Praise for the Books of Jean Carper

"A fascinating volume worth keeping close at hand. . . .
Carper provides scientific evidence, safety factors, descriptions of how each natural remedy, herb, or vitamin works,
and plenty of other pertinent information to enable readers to
draw their own conclusions."
        —*Nashville Banner* on *Miracle Cures*

"Reader-friendly . . . [helps] make sense of the complexity. . . .
Miracle Cures is worth reading for anyone investigating herbs."
        —*USA Today*

"Full of amazing facts and advice. The best of all the books
on the diet-health connection by a long shot, *Food—Your
Miracle Medicine* is everybody's passport to health."
        —John Naisbitt, author of *Megatrends*

"Performs the difficult task of being responsibly informative and highly entertaining at the same time. Open this
book to any page and you will learn something new and
enjoy yourself doing it."
        —*Longevity* on *Food—Your Miracle Medicine*

"*Food—Your Miracle Medicine* is a manifesto for a revolution in mainstream medicine that is happening now."
        —Stephen DeFelice, chairman,
        Foundation for Innovation in Medicine

"Jean Carper, and the increasing number of scientific studies linking a good diet to less disease and sickness that she
reports to the American people, comprise a dynamic consumer movement of great importance."
        —Ralph Nader on *Food—Your Miracle Medicine*

Also by Jean Carper
Food—Your Miracle Medicine
Stop Aging Now!
Miracle Cures

Published by HarperPaperbacks

Jean Carper

The Miracle Heart

The Ultimate Guide to Preventing and Curing Heart Disease with Diet and Supplements

HarperPaperbacks
A Division of HarperCollins*Publishers*

HarperPaperbacks

A Division of HarperCollins*Publishers*

10 East 53rd Street, New York, NY 10022-5299

This book will educate the reader about natural drugs, remedies, treatments, medicines, cures, and "dietary supplements." It is based on the personal experiences, research, and observations of the author, who is not a medical or naturopathic doctor. This book is intended to be informational and by no means should be considered a substitute for advice from a medical or health professional, who should be consulted by the reader in matters relating to his or her health and particularly in respect to any symptoms that may require medical attention. While every effort has been made to ensure that drug selections and dosages are in accordance with current recommendations and practices, because of ongoing research and other factors, the reader is cautioned to check with a health professional about specific recommendations. Anyone with a known disease or serious health condition or who is taking prescription medications should especially seek professional medical advice before taking the natural remedies described in this book. There could be interactions between the natural remedies and other drugs. Also, it should be noted that all dosages discussed in this book apply to adults, not to children, unless otherwise stated. The author and publisher expressly disclaim responsibility for any adverse effects arising from the use or application of the information contained in this book.

ISBN 0-06-101383-8

HarperCollins®, ❦®, and HarperPaperbacks™ are trademarks of HarperCollins Publishers Inc.

First HarperPaperbacks printing: February 2000

Printed in the United States of America

Visit HarperPaperbacks on the World Wide Web at
http://www.harpercollins.com

❖ 10 9 8 7 6 5 4

Contents

Acknowledgments

My ultimate appreciation must go to the pioneering scientists who use their talents, imagination, and energy to investigate with new vigor the astonishing medicinal secrets of food, vitamins, minerals, and other natural remedies. It is their commitment to objective scientific evidence that has boosted the legitimacy of the use of diet and supplements to fight disease, including heart disease. This book is a distillation of their many years of work, creativity, and discovery regarding heart disease. I have read thousands of their research papers and communicated with hundreds of them in personal interviews, on the telephone, by fax, and at conferences. They have given me countless hours of their time, and I thank them profusely.

My most special thanks must go to Janis Jibrin, M.S., R.D., a Washington-based nutritionist who is also a very talented writer and an author in her own right. Janis integrated into this book much new information that is derived from three of my previously published books, *Food—Your Miracle Medicine, Stop Aging Now!,* and *Miracle Cures.* Her meticulous updating of the information in those books and the addition of new research makes *The Miracle Heart* as comprehensive and current as it could be at publication time. Janis has written over one hundred articles for national publications. Her latest book is *The Unofficial Guide to Dieting Safely,* published by Macmillan in 1998. She is coauthor of *Dr. Health'nstein's Body Fun* (Star Press, 1994), an award-winning nutrition education CD-ROM for children.

Introduction

You Can Stop Heart Disease

You probably don't have to look far up the family tree to find someone who has had heart disease, or risk factors for it; it might even be you. Without question, cardiovascular disease is our biggest killer, accounting for more deaths than the next seven leading causes of death combined. Nearly one million Americans die of cardiovascular disease every year—about 2,600 every day or one every thirty-three seconds. Another American will be dead of heart disease by the time you finish reading this page. About 59 million Americans are now living with some form of cardiovascular disease, such as coronary artery disease and high blood pressure that can eventually claim their lives.

The estimated cost of heart disease in 1999: $286.5 billion.

Admittedly, heredity plays a part in a predisposition to heart disease, but biology is far from destiny. There is overwhelming evidence that you can control whether or not you develop heart disease and whether it progresses. Exciting new research confirms daily that you can avoid or overcome heart disease with food and supplements, and that it's never too late to make a difference.

In the last few years new large-scale research studies have made the evidence irrefutable. Even the hardened skeptics have come to agree that the way we eat and the supplements we take not only prevent and reverse risk factors for heart disease such as high blood cholesterol and high blood pressure, but prevent and reverse heart disease itself. Take vitamin E, for example. Some impressive studies looking back on the diet and supplement habits of thousands of people consistently showed that those who took high doses of E were less likely to get heart disease. The tantalizing implication: E protects you from heart disease. Then came the spectacular clincher: a British study giving vitamin E to men who had already had a heart attack. Compared to placebo takers, vitamin E supplementers decreased their risk for a second heart attack by 77 percent! Here in the U.S., the National Institutes of Health–sponsored DASH study showed that eating a diet high in fruits, vegetables, and fiber, and low in sodium, was as effective in lowering blood pressure as medication. These and other compelling studies are all here in this book.

In this book you will discover every scientifically valid dietary substance to forestall or ameliorate heart disease.

The Research Revolution

We are witnessing a marvelous revolution in medicine that emphasizes prevention instead of treatment, and natural ways of treatment as adjuncts to or replacements for conventional medicines. Evidence is piling up, showing how such natural remedies can fight heart disease. Prestigious medical journals are full of reports documenting the awesome powers, unimagined a decade or so ago, of foods and natural supplements to combat high blood pressure, cholesterol, and heart attacks. The evidence comes from such mainstream institutions as Harvard, the University of California, Tufts, Johns Hopkins, Stanford, and Yale, among many.

The anti–heart disease powers of some of the substances now being tested have been suspected for centuries, some for only a few years. Some of the names are familiar, such as vitamin E and C. Others are less so, like coenzyme Q-10, but are now emerging as superstars in the laboratories of scientists trying to prevent and reverse heart disease.

You'll notice throughout this book that one of the most important ways these natural remedies protect your heart is by fighting off free radicals—destructive molecules formed in the body and taken in via environmental pollutants. Free radicals attack circulating blood cholesterol, priming it so it can clog arteries leading to the heart and brain. Antioxidants in foods and supplements neutralize free radicals, putting them out of business. Much heart disease can be chalked up to a global antioxidant deficiency, pitted against an environment, both internally and externally rich in free radicals. Thus, many antioxidant substances such as vitamin E, vitamin C, and coenzyme Q-10 may all work individually and together to prevent heart disease.

Heart-Saving Superfoods

You can eat your way out of an antioxidant deficiency. Foods are chemical concoctions of awesome complexity that enter your cells, altering their composition and dictating their activity. Although you may not think of them as such, foods are potent packages of pharmacological agents that control the behavior of your cells. What you give your cells can make them fortresses filled with armies of antioxidants to resist the ravages of time and free radical attacks that cause heart disease. Or you can provide foods devoid of antioxidants, allowing wholesale massacres and mutilation of your cells—diminishing your prospects for heart disease prevention and longevity. It's mainly the plant foods that are protective: fruits, vegetables, legumes, grains, and oils. Besides having antioxidant powers, these foods fend off heart disease in many other ways: helping reduce blood pressure, and lowering levels of cholesterol and of another heart stopper, homocysteine.

Heart-Saving Supplements

While diets rich in fruits, vegetables, whole grains, and fish are being vigorously investigated for their heart benefits, so are individual vitamins, minerals, and other beneficial compounds in these foods. This represents an earthquake-like shift in the medical view of vitamin supplements. No longer do scientists see vitamins and minerals as just the mundane stuff in

foods that builds strong bones and corrects deficiencies such as scurvy. "We are opening up a whole new
frontier for vitamins," says vitamin investigator Dr.
Ishwarlal Jialal, associate professor of internal medicine and clinical nutrition at the University of Texas
Southwestern Medical Center at Dallas. In the new
order of things, certain key vitamins in doses exceeding those in food promise protection against heart disease far beyond all previous expectations.

As you'll see in this book, the accumulating evidence is staggering.

The case for taking vitamins and minerals and other
supplements to prevent and ameliorate heart disease
grows so persuasive that not taking them is an invita-
tion to reckless aging and premature heart disease. For
instance:

- Heart disease victims have comparatively low
  blood-tissue levels of dietary antioxidants,
  including vitamin E, vitamin C, beta carotene,
  and selenium.
- A deficiency in certain B vitamins can trigger
  artery damage and heart attack; replenishing
  the vitamins often prevents or remedies these
  problems.
- You can't rely on the government-sanctioned
  recommended modest doses of vitamins and
  minerals (RDAs) to combat the ravages of
  heart disease to the maximum, although sometimes even small amounts can prevent or
  reverse deterioration.

Take This Book to Heart

In this book you'll find the latest, most comprehensive research on how to use diet and supplements to prevent, treat, and even reverse heart disease. Essentially, this book brings together my writings on heart disease and nutrition from three previously published books—*Food—Your Miracle Medicine*, *Stop Aging Now!*, and *Miracle Cures*. The research has been updated and new information added to present the most current advice available on the remarkable heart-healing powers of food, vitamins, minerals, and natural remedies, based on hundreds of research studies published in top-notch medical journals and interviews with many of those researchers.

Here's a preview of what you'll find:

- Foods to help fight or reverse your specific condition, whether it's heart disease, high blood cholesterol/triglycerides, high blood pressure, narrowed arteries, or blood clots.
- Vitamins and minerals that combat heart disease, and their specific recommended dosages.
- Herbal and natural remedies that really work—some as well as medications—to keep your heart healthy and allow you to continue an active lifestyle.

Heart disease is our country's most devastating illness, claiming more lives than any other killer. Remember, you are not powerless against it. Armed with the information in this book, you can take control and prevent it, reverse it, or lessen your symptoms. You can stop heart disease. It makes sense to start now.

The DisHEARTening Facts

Unfortunately, the typical American diet and our increasingly sedentary lifestyles have made heart disease an epidemic. Cardiovascular disease (CVD) is the number one killer of Americans.

- About 59 million Americans have one or more types of cardiovascular disease.
- In 1996 (the latest year for which statistics are available) 959,227 died of cardiovascular disease, accounting for 41 percent of all deaths, or one of every 2.4 deaths.
- More than 2,600 Americans die each day of cardiovascular disease, an average of one death every thirty-three seconds.
- Cardiovascular disease claims more lives each year than the next seven leading causes of death combined.
- About one-sixth of those killed by cardiovascular disease are under age 65.
- More women die of heart disease than men; in 1996 women accounted for 52.7 percent of cardiovascular disease deaths; men, 47.3 percent.

- About 52 percent of American adults have total blood cholesterol levels of 200 mg/dL or higher. (After 200 mg/dL, risk for heart disease goes up.)
- Twenty percent of American adults have high total cholesterol (240 mg/dL or more).
- After age 50, women's cholesterol is higher than men's.
- Stroke killed 157,991 people in 1995 (the latest available statistics) and is the third-largest cause of death.
- Stroke is the leading cause of disability in the U.S.
- In 1995, 61 percent of stroke victims were women.

(Source: Statistics adapted from the American Heart Association's 1999 statistical reports.)

Part 1

What to Eat to Fight Heart Disease

If you're afraid of heart disease—and who isn't in a land where it claims nearly a million lives a year?—one of the biggest clues to your survival is knowing what those people eat who don't get heart disease or die of it. Of course, genes and gender are partly at fault. So is lifestyle—smoking, exercise, and stress. But even when scientists eliminate all those things, diet still pops out as vital to whether your arteries clog or your heart gives out. Curbing the progression of artery disease in the first place—it invariably advances with age—is foremost in warding off heart attacks and strokes. But remarkable new evidence shows that even if you ate recklessly in earlier days, and even if you have already had heart problems, including a heart attack, changing your diet now may prevent future cardiac catastrophe and even halt or reverse arterial damage, helping restore arteries to health. It is not too early or too late.

How Arteries Get Clogged and How Food Can Stop It

At birth your arteries are clean, open, and elastic. But early in life the process of artery clogging, known as atherosclerosis or coronary artery disease, begins. Fatty streaks appear in and under the layer of cells that line artery walls. Gradually the streaks are transformed into plaques—fatty scar tissue that bulges into the artery opening, partly choking off blood flow. If one of these plaques breaks down, the clotting mechanism may be triggered. If the clot becomes large enough, it can block blood flow, suffocating large patches of cardiac muscle, an event known as a heart attack. Reduced blood flow can also trigger abnormal heart rhythms—tachycardia and fibrillation—sometimes causing sudden death. Or if a blood vessel to the brain closes off or ruptures, you suffer a stroke.

What you eat is a major determinant of how quickly and severely your arteries get clogged. The right diet can help keep vessels open, free of hazardous clots and flexible enough to serve as healthy conduits for blood flow. Food does this by combating the buildup of cholesterol and other blood fats, and most of all, by affecting blood-clotting factors. Here's what people eat who don't get heart disease, as confirmed by investigators around the world.

Chapter 1

The Foods Your Heart Likes Best

> **Foods That Can Save Arteries and Prevent Heart Disease:** Seafood • Fruits • Vegetables • Nuts • High-Fiber Foods • Magnesium-Rich Foods • Grains • Legumes • Onions • Garlic • Olive Oil • Alcohol in Moderation • Foods High in Vitamin C and E and Beta Carotene

Fish:
The Universal Heart Medicine

The best way to slash your chances of heart disease is, above all, to eat fish, particularly fatty fish, overflowing with omega-3 fatty acids. The evidence of fish's preventive and therapeutic powers against cardiovascular disease is compelling. Seafood's probable main heart medicine is its unique marine fat, so fish may be the one food where fattier is healthier.

Fish with the most good fat: salmon, tuna, mackerel, sardines, herring—fresh, frozen, or canned.

An Ounce a Day

Seafood eaters worldwide have less heart disease and suffer fewer heart attacks. Even eating tiny amounts of fish can have a monumental effect. A landmark Dutch study found that eating, on average, a mere ounce of fish a day cut the chances of fatal heart disease in half. A study at Chicago's Northwestern University Medical School tracking 1,822 men for thirty years found that those who ate the most fish—over an ounce a day—cut their risk of heart disease by about 40 percent and their chance of heart attacks by about half.

A study of 6,000 middle-aged American men revealed that those who ate the marine fat in a one-ounce bite of mackerel or three ounces of bass a day were 36 percent less apt to die of heart disease than men eating less fish. Another twenty-five-year U.S. study of 17,000 men found that fatal heart attacks dropped the more fish they ate. Non-fish eaters had one-third more heart disease deaths than those who ate more than an ounce and a quarter of seafood a day.

If you could look inside people's arteries, you would see that the healthiest ones belong to fish eaters and the most diseased ones to non-fish eaters. As an alternative, you could examine their arteries at autopsy. That's what Danish researchers did recently, and came up with remarkable, unprecedented proof of the power of fish oil to prevent atherosclerosis.

The Danes obtained arteries and fat tissue from forty consecutive autopsies at Frederiksberg Hospital in Denmark. They measured the fish oil in the fat tissue, which revealed how much fatty fish the individual had eaten while alive. Undeniably, the smoothest, cleanest arteries belonged to those with the most omega-3 fat in their tissue—who had eaten the most fish. And the most seriously clogged arteries belonged to those with the least omega-3 fat in their tissue, indicating they had made the mistake of skimping on fatty fish.

Further, new evidence reveals that fish oil, like vitamin C, influences all-important *vascular function*, keeping arteries more relaxed and open so blood can flow through. The omega-3s, like the vitamin, somehow trigger release of nitric oxide, the chemical that tells artery walls to relax.

Fish Prevents Sudden Death

At first, researchers thought fish discouraged heart attacks only by lessening atherosclerosis, the destruction and clogging of arteries. The theory was, fish oil acted as a mild anticoagulant to prevent blood clotting and buildup of plaque that narrows arteries. But exciting new evidence shows that eating fish does much more than previously was thought. It actually protects the muscle of the heart from potentially deadly arrhythmias and cardiac arrest. In short, eating fish can keep you from having a drop-dead heart attack. Indeed, many fish oil authorities, including Harvard emeritus professor of medicine Dr. Alexander Leaf, now believe that regulating heart rhythms is the primary way fish saves lives.

Every year about 250,000 Americans suddenly die when the heart stops because of irregular heart muscle contractions or sudden fibrillation. It can happen without any prior history of heart disease. Recent research finds it happens far less frequently to people who eat fish.

A recent report out of Harvard's long-running Physician's Health Study found that men who ate fish at least once a week had half the risk of sudden cardiac death compared to those eating fish less than once a month. The study tracked 20,551 male physicians aged 40 to 84 years. Incidentally, eating more than one serving of fish weekly didn't mean greater risk reduction, a fact that shows how potent the protection is from such a small amount of fish. In a separate study of more than 800 people living in Washington state, investigators found that those who ate small amounts of fatty fish, such as salmon, herring, and mackerel—even one serving a week— reduced their likelihood of cardiac arrest by a remarkable 50 to 70 percent!

Dr. Leaf explains that fish oil affects the electrical activity and "excitability" of heart cells, just as it does brain cells. In impressive studies, Dr. Leaf has shown that it is much more difficult to induce heart arrhythmias in dogs that are first given fish oil. Indeed, he consistently found it took a 50 percent stronger electrical stimulus to induce cardiac arrhythmias in heart cells that contained high levels of omega-3 fatty acids. Dr. Leaf has new research under way to test the theory in humans. In his new study, patients with implanted defibrillators, who have already had heart attacks, will take either fish oil capsules or a placebo (dummy pill) for a year. The study will reveal whether fish oil reduces the number of times the defibrillator must discharge to correct a heart arrhythmia. Results are due in 2001.

Eating an ounce of fish a day, or a couple of servings a week, slashes your chances of heart attack by one-third to one-half, studies show.

Fish: Heart Attack Survival Food

If you have a heart attack, there's no question about what to do: make a preemptive strike. Get on a high-fish diet immediately. It can cut your chances of future deadly heart attacks by one-third. In fact, eating fish boosts your odds of escaping subsequent heart attacks better than the traditional route of cutting down on foods high in saturated animal fat. So found a ground-breaking two-year study by Michael Burr, M.D., at the Medical Research Council in Cardiff, Wales. Dr. Burr studied 2,033 men who had all had at least one heart attack. He asked one group to eat a five-ounce serving of oily fish, like salmon, mackerel, or sardines, at least twice a week or take fish oil capsules. He instructed a second group to cut down on saturated fatty foods such as butter, cheese, and cream, and a third group to boost fiber intake by eating more bran cereal and whole wheat bread. For comparison, he gave no dietary advice at all to a fourth group.

After two years there was no lifesaving effect from a

low-fat or high-fiber diet. But the impact from eating fish was startling. Deaths among the fish eaters dropped 29 percent! "That's almost fantastic," says Harvard's Dr. Leaf.

In two major studies in England and France, involving about 1,600 heart patients, those who ate omega-3 as fatty fish, fish oil capsules, or canola oil were much less apt to suffer subsequent fatal heart attacks (not necessarily nonfatal heart attacks) than those not taking in high omega-3. In fact, in one study not a single patient on high omega-3s died of cardiac arrest, most likely because of the therapeutic ability of omega-3 fat to suppress fatal arrhythmias after a heart attack.

- **BOTTOM LINE:** If you suffer a heart attack, your odds of having another one go down more if you eat fish twice a week and lots of fruits and vegetables than if you simply follow the conventional advice of cutting down on fat in your diet.

Second Chance After Heart Surgery

If you have a common surgical procedure called balloon angioplasty to open clogged arteries, eating fatty fish may help keep them unclogged. Such arteries tend to clog again in 40 to 50 percent of cases. Yet, some studies—but not all—show that fish oil may cut the chances of reclogging, and may in fact be better than a low-fat diet. Taking fish oil capsules may deter reclosure.

But eating lots of fish may also do the trick, according to a study by Isabelle Bairati, M.D., professor of medicine at Laval University in Quebec City, Canada. She found that consistent fish eating alone before and after surgery kept arteries open just as well as taking fish oil capsules. Those who ate more than eight ounces of seafood a week were roughly half as apt to suffer reclogging after angioplasty as those who ate but a couple of ounces a week. Not surprisingly, fatty fish high in omega-3 fatty acids, like salmon, mackerel, and sardines, were more potent than other kinds.

Ten Ways Fish Oil Fights Heart Disease

1. Blocks platelet aggregation (clotting)
2. Reduces blood vessel constriction
3. Increases blood flow
4. Lowers fibrinogen (clotting factor)
5. Revs up fibrinolytic (clot-dissolving) activity
6. Lowers triglycerides
7. Raises good HDL cholesterol
8. Makes cell membranes more flexible
9. Lowers blood pressure
10. Wards off deadly fibrillation (irregular heartbeats)

How to Choose and Prepare Fish

In the Grocery: Choose fresh fish with bright eyes and firm flesh. Know that canned salmon and tuna are excellent sources of omega-3s. In fact, cheaper canned pink salmon has slightly more omega-3 than red. Choose canned tuna in water to preserve the most omega-3s. Sardines canned in their own oil, labeled sild oil, have the most omega-3s.

At Home: Best way to cook fresh fish: poaching, steaming, sauteing, microwaving. Grilling is okay occasionally, but can create low levels of cancer-causing agents from reactions between high heat and fish protein. Other ways to avoid hazards: Don't eat fish skin, where carcinogens most often reside. Don't eat sport fish, most apt to be unsafe.

Eating Out: Go with broiled, poached, lightly sauteed, or stir-fried fish. Adding fats such as butter, cream, or mayonnaise tends to counteract fish oil's heart benefits. That's also why deep-fried, batter-covered fish is a poor choice. Eating salad dressings made with corn, soybean, and safflower oils along with fish also diminishes its effects. Olive oil and canola are okay.

Garlic Turns Back the Clock on Clogged Arteries

Eating garlic regularly can deter artery clogging, and more remarkably, even reverse the damage, helping heal your arteries, says Arun Bordia, a cardiologist at Tagore

Medical College in India. Dr. Bordia, a pioneering garlic researcher, discovered that feeding garlic to rabbits with 80 percent arterial blockage reduced the degree of blockage, partially restoring the arteries to health.

He then tested garlic on a group of 432 heart disease patients, most recovering from heart attacks. Half the group ate two or three fresh raw or cooked garlic cloves every day for three years. They squeezed the garlic into juice, put it in milk as a "morning tonic," or ate it boiled or minced. The other half ate no garlic. After the first year there was no difference in the rate of heart attacks between the groups.

In the second year, however, deaths among the garlic eaters dropped by 50 percent, and in the third year they sank 66 percent! Nonfatal heart attacks also declined 30 percent the second year and 60 percent the third year. Further, blood pressure and blood cholesterol in the garlic eaters fell about 10 percent. Garlic eaters also had fewer attacks of angina—chest pain. There were no significant cardiovascular changes in the non-garlic eaters.

Dr. Bordia suggests that, over time, steady infusions of garlic both wash away some of the arterial plaque and prevent future damage. Garlic's main weapon is probably a conglomeration of antioxidants. Garlic is said to possess at least fifteen different antioxidants that may neutralize artery-destroying agents.

Note: Cooked garlic was as effective as raw garlic in warding off heart attacks and deaths, according to Dr. Bordia.

A Garlic Bonus. The garlic also produced unexpected health benefits. Dr. Bordia said the garlic eaters reported fewer joint pains, body aches, and asthmatic tendencies; more vigor, energy, and libido; and a better appetite. Particularly impressive was the diminished joint pain in those with osteoarthritis. Five percent dropped out of the study, however, complaining of burning urine, bleeding piles, flatulence, and irritability. Eating raw garlic elicited more complaints than eating it cooked.

Worldwide, eating garlic is linked to less heart disease. A 1981 study of the diets in fifteen countries by researchers at the University of Western Ontario found that those nations with higher garlic consumption had lower rates of heart disease.

Discover the Nutty Heart Drugs

Eat a few nuts a day as an antidote to heart disease, suggests a recent report from Harvard University's famed Nurses Health Study tracking 86,000 women for fourteen years. Women who ate more than five ounces of nuts (all types) a week lowered their chances of heart disease by 35 percent over women who never ate nuts or had no more than an ounce a month. Eating more nuts also meant a 39 percent drop in heart disease deaths and 35 percent lowered risk of a nonfatal heart attack. In another ongoing Harvard study tracking thousands of male physicians, compared to those eating the least nuts, men who ate the most were at lower risk from dying from heart disease.

Theses results are in sync with research done by Gary Fraser, Ph.D., professor of medicine at Loma Linda University in California. In a study of 31,208 Seventh-

Day Adventists, Dr. Fraser found that nuts stood out as the number one food among those who did not suffer heart attacks. Those who munched on nuts at least five times a week had roughly *half the chance of heart attack and coronary death* as those who ate nuts less than once a week. Even snacking on nuts once a week appeared to cut heart disease risk about 25 percent. About 32 percent of the nuts consumed were peanuts, 29 percent almonds, 16 percent walnuts, and 23 percent other nuts.

It's not as zany as it may seem. Nuts are rich in fiber and monounsaturated olive oil type fats, known to counteract heart disease. Nuts are also packed with various antioxidants, including vitamin E, selenium (especially Brazil nuts), and ellagic acid (notably walnuts), that could guard arteries against the ravages of cholesterol. Most nuts are also rich in the amino acid arginine, some of which the body converts to nitric oxide, which relaxes blood vessels and lowers blood pressure. Nitric oxide also discourages blood from becoming "sticky," meaning less chance for clotting.

Since nuts are high in fat, although most is beneficial fat, you can't eat nuts with abandon if you are concerned about weight. In Dr. Fraser's study, however, enthusiastic nut eaters were less obese than non-nut eaters. Dr. Fraser did not determine how many nuts people ate at one time. A sensible amount, depending on a person's weight, would be an ounce or two a day.

The Italian Experiment

What do Italian women eat who do and don't have heart attacks? To find out, Italian investigators at the Instituto di Ricerche Farmacologiche Mario Negri in Milan analyzed the diets of 936 older women.

They found that women who ate the most carrots and fresh fruit had a 60 percent lower chance of heart attack; those who ate the most green vegetables and fish had a 40 percent lower risk. Moderate alcohol consumption also reduced the risk 30 percent, but heavy drinking increased it 20 percent. Women with the highest risk ate more meat, specifically ham and salami, butter, and total fat.

Use Vegetable Power to Block Heart Attacks

Devouring fruits and vegetables can slash your chances of heart attacks and strokes, even if you have already suffered one. Unquestionably, dedicated fruit and vegetable eaters have better arteries. Vegetarians have the lowest rates of cardiovascular disease. Women who ate one additional large carrot or one-half cup of sweet potatoes (or other foods rich in beta carotene) every day slashed their risk of heart attack by 22 percent and stroke by 40 to 70 percent, according to Harvard studies.

For instance, in a Harvard study tracking more than 90,000 female nurses, those eating the most beta carotene (more than 11,000 IU daily) had a 22 percent lower risk of heart disease than women getting less than 3,800 IU daily. The high–beta carotene eaters' risk of stroke was 37 percent lower. In a large-scale multicenter European study, those who took in the least beta carotene were at a 260 percent higher risk of a first heart attack than those who ate the most beta carotene.

Beta carotene may lengthen your life: Men who ate 6 milligrams of beta carotene daily (one carrot) over twenty-five years had a 28 percent lower risk of death from all causes compared with men eating the least beta carotene, reported University of Texas researchers.

Fruits and vegetables are also a good post–heart attack prescription. If you survive a heart attack, eating fruits and vegetables can save you from another cardiac event and death even better than just cutting back on high-fat meats and dairy foods, a recent year-long study of 400 heart attack patients in India found. Doctors put half the heart attack survivors on a standard low-fat diet, the other half on an "experimental" diet heavy on fruits, grains, nuts, legumes, fish, and vegetables. Specifically, the diet called for about fourteen ounces of fruits and vegetables a day. (This included guava, grapes, papaya, bananas, oranges, limes, apples, spinach, radishes, tomatoes, lotus root, mushrooms, onions, garlic, fenugreek seeds, peas, and red beans.)

After a year, the fruit and vegetable eaters had 40 percent fewer cardiac events and 45 percent fewer deaths from all causes than the low-fat eaters. The researchers concluded that if everyone immediately went on a high fruit and vegetable diet after a heart attack, countless lives could be saved.

Important: For best results, a heart attack victim should get on the vegetarian type diet as quickly as possible. In the Indian study, the diet was commenced within seventy-two hours of the attack.

Additionally, a Dutch study of heart patients found that switching to a vegetarian, low-saturated-fat, low-cholesterol diet for two years both halted and reversed arterial damage. The most likely explanation: the vegetable carotenes and other antioxidants in fruits and vegetables help keep arteries unclogged and healthy, say researchers.

Surprise! Tomatoes Fight Heart Disease

Lately scientists are hailing tomatoes because they are packed full of the antioxidant lycopene, thought to help prevent various cancers, including prostate, gastrointestinal, and cervical cancers. Elderly women who function best mentally and physically in old age also have high blood counts of lycopene.

Now there's a big new reason to applaud tomatoes: A major new study by researchers at the University of North Carolina shows that eating tomatoes also fends off heart disease. The study of 1,379 European men found that those who ate the most lycopene (as shown by analyzing lycopene content in body fat) were only half as apt to have a heart attack as men who ate the least lycopene.

Researchers believe the antioxidant activity of lycopene, a red pigment in tomatoes, brings about reduction in heart attacks. Recent tests suggest lycopene is a much more potent antioxidant than beta carotene, and even vitamin E.

You absorb the most lycopene, surprisingly, in cooked or canned tomatoes and tomato products. "You get five times more lycopene from tomato sauce than an equivalent amount of fresh tomatoes," says chief researcher Lenore Kohlmeier.

Best foods sources of lycopene are tomato paste, ketchup, and tomato sauce. Tomatoes ripened on the vine have more lycopene than those that ripen after being picked. A tomato must be red to contain lycopene; green and yellow tomatoes are not good lycopene sources.

Fill Up on Fiber

Bump up your intake of fiber and knock down your risk for heart disease; that's what international research on the subject indicates. For instance, men who ate the most fiber (25 or more grams daily) had one-third fewer heart attacks than men eating the least fiber (12 grams), according to a Harvard study. All types of fiber counted—in fruit, vegetables, cereals, and grains. Increasing daily fiber by 10 grams—as in one cup of shredded wheat and one-half grapefruit—lowers heart attack risk 20 percent, said lead investigator Dr. Eric Rimm.

In addition to fiber's famed blood cholesterol–lowering effects, fiber may "push more fat through the system so that it is not absorbed," suggests Dr. Rimm. That's because soluble fiber—the type in oats, psyllium, beans, and many fruits and vegetables—swells in the intestine and may trap fat and send it out before you can absorb it. (See page 82–83 for a list of foods high in soluble fiber).

- **BOTTOM LINE:** To lower your risk of heart disease and other chronic illnesses, get 25 to 30 grams of fiber daily from a variety of sources including whole grain cereals, beans, fruits, and vegetables. Whole foods are better than fiber supplements because they provide other heart-protective factors.

Greens and Beans: More Magnesium

Evidence pours in that too little magnesium makes you more susceptible to heart disease. A new study of 15,000 men and women, ages 45 to 64, by University of Minnesota researchers found that those with existing cardiovascular disease, high blood pressure, and diabetes had significantly lower blood levels of magnesium than those free of such diseases. Women with low blood levels of magnesium were more apt to have high bad type LDL cholesterol and thickening of the walls of the carotid (neck) arteries, an indication that arteries are clogged. Those with high dietary and blood magnesium had higher good type HDL cholesterol as well as lower levels of blood sugar and insulin, a hormone that damages artery walls.

Best food sources of magnesium: tofu, greens such as spinach and Swiss chard, wheat bran, pumpkin and sunflower seeds, dried beans, oysters, halibut, mackerel, grouper cod, and sole.

Try the Japanese Heart-Saving Diet

Eat like the Japanese used to. With the invasion of westernized high-fat fast food, Japan's heart disease rate is creeping upward. But for years that country's low-fat, high-fish diet was a model for a heart disease–free life. In 1957 Ancel Keys, then a professor at the University of Minnesota, began tracking heart disease rates in seven countries: the United States, Finland, the Netherlands, Italy, Yugoslavia, Greece, and Japan. He discovered that Western countries generally had five times more fatal heart disease than Japan, which had the lowest of all. For example, eastern Finland had the most heart disease, about eight times more than Japan. Striking was the fact that the Japanese ate only 9 percent of calories in fat with only 3 percent from animal fat, whereas the Finns' diet was 39 percent fat with 22 percent from animal fat.

Although the classic heart-saving Japanese diet is disappearing, University of Helsinki researchers recently interviewed Japanese villagers who said they still followed the traditional diet of their ancestors. This is what they ate on an average day: four to five cups of rice, five to eight ounces of fruit, about nine ounces of vegetables, two ounces of beans, about two ounces of meat, three to four ounces of fish, one-half cup of milk, one egg or less, two teaspoons of sugar, one and one-half tablespoons of soy sauce. The men also drank fifteen ounces of beer, the women only a trace of beer.

Thus, the classic Japanese diet is low in calories, fat, and meat, and high in fish, fruit, vegetables, and rice. The one blot on the diet is excessive sodium, largely from soy sauce, which is partially blamed for their high rate of strokes. If you restrict the sodium, eating as the Japanese once did seems an excellent way to escape heart disease.

Why Mediterranean Hearts Are Stronger

For a better heart, adopt the diet of people who live around the Mediterranean Sea, particularly in Greece, Italy, Spain, and southern France. Such people are only half as likely to die of heart disease as Americans. Indeed, some researchers are convinced the Mediterranean diet is a more agreeable way for Americans to save their hearts than is a lower-fat diet, generally advocated by health officials. No, the Mediterranean diet is not low-fat; in fact, Mediterraneans typically eat more fat than Americans do. But there is a big difference. About three-fourths of all their fat calories come from monounsaturated fat, exemplified by olive oil; they also eat very little saturated animal fat. For example, residents of the island of Crete sometimes drink olive oil by the glass, running up their quota of calories from fat to over 40 percent. Yet, Dr. Ancel Keys found in his landmark Seven Countries Study that Cretans rarely succumbed to heart disease. In a fifteen-year period only 38 out of 10,000 Cretans died of heart disease, compared with 773 Americans, giving the United States twenty times as much deadly heart disease as Crete. Other Mediterranean populations also had low rates.

The clincher: In stringent tests, the Mediterranean diet has proven superior to the "Western" low-fat diet in saving heart attack victims from having another one. In the first study in 1994, Michel de Lorgeril, M.D., and colleagues at INSERM, the French equivalent of our National Institutes of Health, found that the risk of having another heart attack or dying was about 70 percent lower in a group of 605 heart attack survivors who ate a Mediterranean diet for twenty-seven months rather than a typical low-fat diet recommended by U.S. government authorities and the American Heart Association.

In a 1999 study, the results were nearly identical. Individuals who ate a Mediterranean diet for nearly four years were 50 to 70 percent less apt to suffer a repeat heart attack than those on a low-fat "Western" diet.

How to Eat the Mediterranean Way

Eat Lots of Fruits, Vegetables, Grains, Beans, and Nuts: These hearty complex carbohydrates are the mainstay of the Mediterranean diet. Fruits and vegetables are packed with antioxidants, including vitamin C and beta carotene, that seem to help deter artery clogging and prevent heart attacks. Grains and beans are particularly rich in cholesterol-lowering and disease-fighting fiber. That includes pasta, rice, couscous, bulgur wheat, and polenta (cornmeal). Nuts are good protein substitutes, full of nutrients and antioxidants. And don't forget garlic; it's a daily staple in Mediterranean cuisine. To eat the Mediterranean way, most Americans must at least double the amount of fruits, vegetables, bread, pasta, and other grains they typically eat.

Restrict Meat, Eat Fish: The Mediterranean diet is largely plant-based. However, it is not vegetarian. You can eat standard servings of red meat (beef, pork, lamb, veal) a few times a month or red meat in smaller amounts more often—but no more than an average of one ounce a day, says Harvard researcher Frank Sacks, M.D., an advocate of the Mediterranean diet. Okay are four to six ounces of poultry three or four times a week, and four to six ounces of fish three to seven times a week. In fact, fish is recommended. In the latest French study of heart attack survivors, those who ate fish best warded off a subsequent heart attack. Those with higher blood levels of omega-3 type fish oil were less apt to have a recurrent heart attack or other cardiovascular problem. In studies, red meat has been linked to cancer; in contrast, fish, especially the oil in fatty fish such as salmon and sardines, has been tied to less heart disease and cancer, and greater longevity.

Eat Olive Oil, Curb Other Fats: The main source of fat in the Mediterranean diet is olive oil— two to three tablespoons a day. Olive oil lowers bad LDL blood cholesterol, but not good HDL cholesterol. Unlike corn oil, olive oil is not easily oxidized, thus does not spew off free radicals—chemicals that damage cells, promoting chronic diseases. In fact, olive oil seems to actively protect arteries; research shows it has antioxidant activity and helps curb high insulin and blood sugar levels that destroy arteries.

Eaters of a Mediterranean diet also consume very little omega-6 type fat—or hydrogenated fats and trans fats, found to be so detrimental to the heart and arteries.

Important: Substitute olive oil for other fats such as butter, margarine, mayonnaise. Topping off an already high-fat diet with olive oil can add dangerous pounds. Olive oil, like other oils, has 120 calories per tablespoon. "If you fill up on fat, including olive oil, you'll just get fat." says William Castelli, M.D., former director of the Framingham (Massachussetts) Heart Study.

A final word about fat: The Mediterranean diet ranges in fat from 25 percent of calories in southern Italy to 40 percent of calories from fat in Crete, most of it from olive oil and very little from saturated animal fat. Says Harvard's Walter Willett, "The type of fat is more important than total fat." He calls larger percentages of calories from olive oil, unlike other fats, safe and beneficial if you are active and don't have a weight problem.

Go Easy on Eggs, Cheese, and Sweets: The Mediterranean diet includes few eggs—no more than one egg a week, including those in baked goods. You can eat small portions of preferably low-fat and non-fat yogurt (a cup) and cheese (half to one ounce) every day. For example, grate Parmesan over pasta and crumble feta cheese over salads. You can eat *dolci*, as the Italians call sweets, such as cookies and cake rich in sugar and saturated fat, a few times a week. The traditional Mediterranean dessert is fresh fruit.

Drink Wine in Moderation—If You Wish: A glass or two of wine a day with meals is optional on the Mediterranean diet. Numerous studies suggest that wine, notably red wine, may discourage artery clogging and heart disease.

Caution: Don't take up drinking alcohol as a health measure; if you do drink alcohol, be moderate—a glass of wine a day for women, two daily glasses for men. Too much alcohol is a far greater health hazard than not drinking at all. Don't drink if you are pregnant or if drinking puts yourself or others at risk.

How to Buy and Prepare
Food the Mediterranean Way

At the Market: Buy fresh seasonal produce; restrict processed foods. If you cannot get good vine-ripened tomatoes, buy canned whole tomatoes, preferably plum tomatoes, which have more flavor than typical supermarket tomatoes picked when green. Choose bread that is dense, heavy, chewy, now available at many supermarkets and specialty bakeries. If you are unfamiliar with olive oil, start out with lighter, less robust brands and work up to the stronger flavored types. The more fragrant the oil, the less you need use for taste. Buy strongly flavored cheese, such as Parmesan, so you can get the taste with less.

At the Table: Drizzle olive oil on bread or toast or use bread to sop up juices from the plate. Don't use butter or margarine. If you drink wine with meals, sip it slowly, don't guzzle it down on an empty stomach. Begin each meal with a salad dressed lightly with olive oil and lemon juice, as they do in Mediterranean countries. Put a big bowl of fresh fruit on the table (oranges, peaches, pears, figs, pears, grapes, apples) for dessert, and individual knives (except for young children) for peeling or cutting it up.

In the Kitchen: Prepare fish simply by broiling, grilling, or poaching. For sauteing vegetables, use less expensive olive oil; use good quality, fragrant extra-virgin olive oil for salads, sauces, and on bread. Instead of covering vegetables with butter and margarine, use a little olive oil, dash of lemon juice, salt and pepper. Instead of using meat as the centerpiece of a meal, combine smaller pieces of meat, poultry, and fish with pasta, rice, and a combination of vegetables. Add fresh or canned tuna fish to tomato pasta sauces, for example.

Eating Out: Ask for less cheese on your pizza and more tomato sauce and vegetables, including garlic, onions, peppers. Choose tomato sauces for pasta rather than high-fat cream sauces. Ask for grilled or broiled fish without sauces or with sauces on the side. Ask for olive oil instead of butter, and fresh fruit for dessert—chances are the chef has some in the kitchen even if it is not on the menu. Ask for olive oil and lemon to make your own dressing if it is not otherwise available on salads.

Foods Highest in Artery-Protecting Monos
Percentage of fat as monounsaturated

Hazelnuts	81
Avocados	80
Olive oil	72
Almonds	71
Canola oil	60

- **BOTTOM LINE:** A relatively high-fat diet is not hazardous to the heart if it is very low in animal fat and high in olive oil type fat. Harvard nutritionists favor a Mediterranean-style diet with 35 to 40 percent of fat calories, mostly in monounsaturated fat, over the more restrictive 30-percent-of-calories-in-fat diet widely recommended by government heart officials.

Eat Olive Oil: The Heart-Safe Fat

In Dr. Keys's study, the most enthusiastic consumers of olive oil type fat among the Mediterranean peoples were least likely to die of cancer or anything else! Using "monos" as the major source of fat was the only dietary factor, according to Dr. Keys, that warded off death from all causes. No wonder olive oil is sometimes called the "longevity food."

What makes monounsaturated fat, dominant in olive oil, better for the heart? Chemically, it is simply nicer to arteries. It lowers bad LDL cholesterol, but not good HDL cholesterol. Additionally, monounsaturated fat has antioxidant activity that fends off artery damage from LDL cholesterol. In Italy, physicians have used olive oil as therapy after heart attacks. They find that such patients have better blood profiles, making them less vulnerable to future heart attacks. Further, Harvard's Dr. Walter Willett says, there are "centuries of epidemiological evidence about the benefits of olive oil."

Another reason olive oil is close to the hearts of health authorities: nobody has found any danger in it. "It's the only really safe fat," insists Harry Demopoulos, M.D., a New York researcher on antioxidants. Monounsaturated fat is also concentrated in almond, hazelnut, canola, and avocado oils.

Note: Extra virgin, cold-pressed olive oil is best.

"In the [Mediterranean diet] olive oil is a major source of energy, fat averages 35 to 40 percent of total calories, and rates of coronary disease are as low as in populations with very low-fat diets."
                                    —Frank Sacks, M.D.,
                          Harvard School of Public Health

Eight Ways to the Med Diet

Here's how to turn your typical American diet into a Mediterranean type diet:

1. Double your seafood intake.
2. Increase vegetable consumption by 66 percent and fruit by 10 percent.
3. Eat 20 percent more whole grains and beans.
4. Eat 45 percent less red meat.
5. Eat 16 percent fewer eggs.
6. Eat four times as much olive oil.
7. Eat half as much of other vegetable oils.
8. Eat 50 percent less whole milk, cream, and butterfat.

Sure Way to Poison Arteries

Animal fat is the primary dietary demon in heart disease. It destroys arteries by raising blood cholesterol, encouraging blood stickiness, and suppressing clot-dissolving mechanisms, leaving arteries clogged and constricted. Populations who eat a lot of animal fat have the highest rates of coronary heart disease in the world. And as intake of animal fat goes up, so does heart disease. A 1990 World Health Organization report observes that populations eating from 3 to 10 percent of their total calories in animal fat have little heart disease. Eating more saturated fat brings on "marked and progressive" fatal heart disease. In the United States and other Western countries, saturated fat often accounts for a deadly 15 to 20 percent of calories.

Other good news: You can reverse your mistakes and help unclog arteries by giving up animal fat. Several studies show that restricting fat, namely animal fat, can help block formation and growth of fatty deposits that clog arteries and may even help shrink such fatty buildup. David H. Blankenhorn, M.D., at the University of Southern California School of Medicine, who found such a low-fat diet (5 percent of calories in saturated fat) successful in coronary bypass patients, said most people can save their arteries from animal-fat destruction by simply "substituting low-fat dairy products for high-fat dairy products."

"If I had to tell people just one thing to lower their risk of heart disease, it would be to reduce their intake of foods of animal origin, specifically animal fats, and to replace those fats with complex carbohydrates—grains, fruits and vegetables."

—Ernst Schaefer, M.D.,
USDA Human Nutrition
Research Center on Aging
at Tufts University

A Tot a Day Keeps the Doctor Away

Drink alcohol moderately, if you drink. A drink or two a day may discourage heart disease, suggests dozens of studies. One study declared two-drink-a-day imbibers 40 percent less likely than nondrinkers to be hospitalized for heart attacks. The largest study on alcohol consumption ever done, involving nearly half a million middle-aged and elderly Americans, recently found that those who consumed one drink a day had a 20 percent lower overall death rate than nondrinkers. Further, death from all cardiovascular disease (heart disease, stroke, and other circulatory diseases), more likely after age 60, was 30 to 40 percent lower among one-a-day imbibers, said lead researcher Michael J. Thun, M.D., of the American Cancer Society.

A major 1991 study by Eric Rimm at the Harvard University School of Public Health showed that men who averaged one-half to one drink a day had 21 percent less coronary artery disease than abstainers. One to one-and-a-half daily drinks shaved 32 percent off their heart disease odds. Heavier drinking might depress heart disease odds even further, but the problem is more than two drinks a day puts you in high risk territory for two other diseases.

"The maximum safe dose of alcohol is two drinks a day," says William Castelli, M.D., former director of the Framingham Heart Study. Studies consistently find, he says, that the risk of heart disease falls slightly with one to two daily drinks, but that your chances of death from all causes, including cancer, rise with three drinks a day. One study showed that three to five alcoholic drinks a day increased death rates 50 percent.

After reviewing some three dozen studies, British researcher Richard Doll, M.D., emeritus professor of medicine at Oxford University, agreed the facts are clear: drinking small to moderate amounts of alcohol during middle and old age "reduces the risk of premature death," pushing down deaths from vascular disease by about one-third. However, alcohol is not likely to reduce mortality in those under age 45, he says. Indeed, drinking increases death rates from cirrhosis, injuries, and violence in younger people. Also, alcohol benefits men more, because women have less heart disease and are more vulnerable to alcohol-related liver damage and breast cancer; the risk of breast cancer rises about 10 percent per extra drink per day, says Doll.

Can you drink after a heart attack? Yes, if you don't overdo it. In fact, light or moderate drinking of alcohol—two to six drinks per week—may benefit heart disease survivors, but heavy drinking definitely is harmful, according to a Harvard study of 5,000 men with a history of heart disease. Compared with nondrinkers, the greatest drop in death risk—down 27 percent—came in men who drank two to four drinks per week. One drink a day cut death odds by 21 percent. Drinking more did not further cut cardiovascular deaths.

Some possible reasons for alcohol's heart benefits: alcohol boosts good type HDL cholesterol; wine, notably red wine, is an anticoagulant and discourages dangerous oxidation of bad LDL cholesterol; alcohol can relieve stress, alcoholic beverages contain antioxidants, and alcohol has anti-inflammatory activity.

"There is no other drug that is so efficient [at preventing heart attacks] as the moderate intake of alcohol."

—*Serge Renaud, M.D.,*
former researcher at INSERM,
France's medical research
institution similar to our
National Institutes of Health

Stout-Hearted Frenchmen— Is It the Wine?

Given the choice of an alcoholic beverage for the heart and health in general, it probably should be red wine, a medicine dating back more than four thousand years. According to R. Curtis Ellison, M.D., chief of the Department of Preventive Medicine and Epidemiology at the Boston University School of Medicine, research suggests wine reduces cardiovascular disease better than distilled spirits or beer. Much evidence for the benefits of red wine comes from France.

Curiously, Frenchmen have one-third as many heart attacks as American men, even though the French indulge in fatty foods and have cholesterol and blood pressure as high as American men. This so-called French paradox, some scientists suggest, is explained by the French habit of drinking wine, especially red wine, with meals. Dr. Alun Evans, of Queens University in Belfast, notes that Frenchmen have one-third fewer heart attacks than Irishmen. Both drink the same amount of alcohol, but there's one big difference, he says. The French drink mainly wine; the Irish drink more hard liquor.

Red wine appears superior to white wine in fighting heart disease. For starters, in most of the studies showing wine's protective effects, the wine has been red. Red wine is loaded with more antioxidants than white, and there is even some evidence that white wine may promote artery damage. Red wine contains high amounts of flavonoids that have anticoagulant activity. Thus, French health authorities suggest that wine consumed along with fatty meals *counteracts* the fat hazard. Fatty foods tend to make the blood more sluggish so it is apt to clot and plug up arteries. Wine may thwart that process. The scientists caution the wine drinking should be regular and "moderate—no more than two to three four-ounce glasses of wine a day."

Drinking wine, notably red wine, in moderation may even extend your life, mostly by lessening heart disease, says leading French scientist Serge C. Renaud. In recent research, he tracked 34,000 middle-aged French men for ten to fifteen years; about three-fourths drank wine, primarily red wine, usually with meals.

Dr. Renaud's findings: Men drinking two to three glasses of wine daily had a 30 percent reduction in death rates from all causes compared with non-drinkers or occasional drinkers. Caution: heavy drinkers had a 40 percent higher death rate. Most of the lifesaving value of wine was focused on the heart. Moderate drinkers were 35 percent less apt to die of cardiovascular disease. Surprisingly, moderate drinkers also had an 18 to 24 percent drop in deaths from all cancers. (However, other research finds that alcohol can boost the odds of breast, oral cavity, and liver cancers. More than four drinks a day triples breast cancer risk, for example.)

Dr. Renaud says the new study adds to the evidence that the French paradox is partly due to the regular consumption of wine.

- **BOTTOM LINE:** If you already drink and have no problems with alcohol, one drink a day for women and two drinks a day for men on a regular basis may help protect your heart. More alcohol is dangerous, and binge drinking is particularly harmful to your heart and general health. And alcohol, even in moderation, may raise breast cancer risk, so those with a history of breast cancer should not take up drinking. If you don't drink, do not take up drinking as a way to prevent cardiovascular disease. And if you are a heavy drinker, cut down. Alcohol in heavy doses is definitely a heart poison, capable of inducing severe heart damage and sudden death.

Drink Purple Grape Juice

If you don't drink alcohol, consider drinking purple grape juice instead. It may cut heart disease risk as well as red wine does. Georgetown University researchers found that putting blood platelets in purple grape juice blocked mechanisms leading to blood clots and heart attacks. Platelets in the grape juice were 30 percent less likely to clot; they also released three times more nitric oxide, a chemical that dilates blood vessels and blocks clot-promoting platelet stickiness.

Dr. John Folts as the University of Minnesota also found that purple grape juice has artery-protecting anticoagulant activity. In his studies, three ounces of purple grape juice had as much blood-thinning activity as one ounce of red wine. That means it takes fifteen ounces of purple grape juice to equal the anticoagulant activity of an ordinary five-ounce glass of red wine. Researchers credit antioxidant flavonoids, the pigments mainly in grape skins and seeds, as the active ingredients. White wine and white grape juice are ineffective because they contain low levels of colorful flavonoids.

New research at Tufts University finds that bottled purple grape juice has high antioxidant capacity—four times that of orange and apple juice.

- **BOTTOM LINE:** If you don't drink alcohol, or even if you do, have two cups of purple grape juice daily.

Does Coffee Promote Heart Disease?

There's scant evidence that you need to give up coffee or caffeine to save your heart, although it seems wise for some people at high risk of heart disease to restrict their intake. A 1992 analysis of eleven major studies on the subject by Martin G. Myers, M.D., of the University of Toronto found no link between coffee consumption and heart disease whether subjects drank one cup or more than six cups a day. Similarly, the long-running Harvard study tracking about 86,000 women for ten years found that coffee did not increase heart disease risk, even at six or more cups daily.

On the other hand, a ten-year follow-up study of more than 100,000 individuals by Kaiser Permanente's Dr. Klatsky suggested that four or more cups of coffee a day boosted heart disease chances about 30 percent in men and up to 60 percent in women. There was no danger in tea, suggesting caffeine is not the culprit. Dr. Klatsky advises individuals at high risk of heart disease to limit coffee intake to less than four cups a day. Another recent study found that drinking ten or more cups of coffee a day tripled the risk of heart disease.

And coffee may raise blood levels of the artery-damaging amino acid homocysteine; high levels are linked to heart disease. In Norway heavy drinkers—nine cups a day—of caffeinated coffee, but not decaf, had 25 percent higher homocysteine, researchers found, which could raise heart disease risk up to 20 percent. On the other hand, caffeinated black tea drinkers had lower homocysteine, possibly because tea contains folic acid. This may help explain why some studies have linked coffee drinking to more heart disease and tea to less.

"For people drinking up to six cups of coffee a day there is no strong reason to give it up, and particularly, no strong reason to switch to decaf."
— *Walter Willett, M.D.,*
Harvard School of Public Health

What to Eat if You Have Chest Pain (Angina)

Chest pain, or angina, is a warning sign that arteries are getting too narrow or partially blocked so oxygen and blood cannot flow through easily. Such narrowing is usually due to atherosclerosis, an accumulation of plaque in the coronary arteries that take oxygen to the heart muscle. It also can result from heart spasms.

Chest pain is linked to low blood levels of the antioxidants vitamin E, vitamin C, and beta carotene—and omega-3 fish oil. Thus, to alleviate angina, eat more fruits, vegetables, oily fish, cereals, nuts, and vegetable oils rich in vitamin E, advises researcher Rudolph A. Riemersma, M.D., at the University of Edinburgh. In a major study of 500 middle-aged men—half with angina—Dr. Riemersma found chest pain least likely in those with higher-than-average blood levels of carotene, vitamin C, and particularly vitamin E. Indeed, men with the lowest blood levels of vitamin E were two and a half times more likely to suffer angina than those with the highest levels of vitamin E. Presumably, the vitamin's antioxidant activity discourages arterial damage and clogging. In further research, Dr. Riemersma found that men with higher blood platelet levels of one type of fish oil, known as EPA, were similarly protected from angina.

Irregular Heartbeats: Is Coffee a Cause?

If you suffer from arrhythmias—irregular heartbeats—it seems wise to restrict caffeine, but you may not need to give it up entirely. Dr. Martin G. Myers, at the University of Toronto, analyzed twenty-three recent studies on the connection between caffeine and heart arrhythmia, and found no evidence that less than 500 milligrams of caffeine—about five cups of coffee a day—increased the frequency or severity of cardiac arrhythmias in normal persons or in patients with heart problems.

Still, some experts think it a good idea to drink only a couple of cups of coffee a day if you have irregular heartbeats. Harvard investigator Thomas B. Graboys gave subjects with life-threatening ventricular arrhythmias caffeine tablets comparable to drinking two cups of coffee and then had them pedal stationary bicycles for five minutes every hour for three hours. Their heart rhythms did not change, whether they had taken the caffeine or placebo pills. Dr. Graboys says, "To categorically proscribe all caffeine for someone with arrhythmia doesn't make sense. There's no reason they can't have one or two cups of coffee."

On the other hand, high doses of caffeine, as found in nine or ten cups of coffee, can aggravate preexisting ventricular arrhythmias. Further, heartbeat irregularities may be exaggerated in individuals particularly sensitive to caffeine. Recent research at the Oregon Health Sciences University found that the amount of caffeine in two and a half cups of coffee more easily induced severe ventricular arrhythmias in a select population of "caffeine sensitive" individuals. To be extra safe, they advise heart disease patients to limit coffee to two cups a day.

"At three or more drinks [of alcohol] a day, you don't see adverse coronary effects, but you do see increases in high blood pressure, cirrhosis of the liver, throat cancer, accidents, hospitalizations and mortality."

—Arthur L. Klatsky, *chief of cardiology,*
Kaiser Permanente Medical Center,
Oakland, California

Holiday Heart Syndrome

Can alcohol cause heartbeat disturbances? Decidedly yes, whether you are an alcoholic or casual drinker, say authorities. Alcohol-induced arrhythmias frequently cause sudden cardiac death among alcoholics.

It's so common, for example, in emergency rooms to see people with severe arrhythmias after alcoholic binges on weekends and holidays, particularly between Christmas Eve and New Year's Day, that the problem has been dubbed "holiday heart syndrome." This type of fibrillation or flutter usually vanishes when the alcohol effects wear off, leaving no signs of permanent heart damage. Although it's more common among alcoholics or longtime heavy drinkers, holiday heart syndrome can also strike occasional or moderate drinkers who embark on a drinking binge.

Clearly, heavy drinking boosts your chances of cardiac arrest as well as stroke. One study found that 40 percent of women who suffered sudden death were diagnosed as alcoholics. According to the well-known Framingham Heart Study, persons who consumed more than five or six drinks a day were more likely to die of sudden death even though they did not show signs of coronary artery disease.

The longer and harder you drink, the more susceptible you are to cardiovascular damage. Cutting down on alcohol consumption often diminishes arrhythmia.

Drop Pounds, Drop Heart Disease Odds

Getting fat, especially if that fat tends to park on your belly, means a higher likelihood of developing heart disease. Being overweight ushers in major risk factors for heart disease such as high blood cholesterol, diabetes, and high blood pressure. Fortunately, losing weight, even as little as 5 to 10 percent of your body weight (10 pounds for many people) usually gets rid of these conditions and brings down your risk.

A recent study of thousands of people drawn from the famed Framingham study and a huge government health survey tracks the rise in heart disease risk with increasing body weight. The study examined the lifetime risk of developing coronary heart disease for people 45 to 54 years old. Men who were not obese faced a 35 percent chance of developing the disease in their lifetime; a 25 percent chance for nonobese women. For the mildly obese, risk inched up to 38 percent for men, 29 percent for women; then up to 42 percent and 32 percent for moderately obese men and women. But severe obesity raised risk to 46 percent for men and 37 percent for women. In this study, "not obese" meant a BMI of 22.5, and BMIs of 27.5, 32.5, and 37.5 marked mild, moderate, and severe obesity. (See box on page 52 for definition of BMI.)

Anyone who's tried to lose weight and keep it off knows it's not easy. While there's no one proven formula for success, to increase your chances, find a program that emphasizes a balanced diet, exercise, and includes a behavioral/psychological component. Set modest goals; for instance, aim to lose 10 pounds over one to three months. Maintain that weight for a while before attempting to lose more. Eating a diet rich in fruits, vegetables, and whole grains and low in saturated fat will help you shed those pounds and develop the good habits that will keep weight down for good.

What Is Obesity?

What exactly is obesity? Scientists are still arguing over the definition, but at least they're starting to use a common measure in their debates. It's called Body Mass Index (BMI), a calculation that describes relative weight for height (see table on next page). A government-sponsored expert panel on obesity recently took a crack at the definition, deeming "overweight" a BMI of 25 to 29.9; "obese" a BMI of 30 or above.

By these standards, 97 million American adults—55 percent of the population—are considered overweight or obese. Many obesity experts, including ex-surgeon general C. Everett Koop, who now heads Shape Up America!, criticized the new guidelines, saying they are unnecessarily stringent and may discourage those who have a hard time making it down to a BMI of under 25. Previous definitions were more generous; the National Center for Health Statistics defined overweight as a BMI of 28 for men and 27 for women.

Remember, the BMI chart is not infallible. Although BMI gets closer to measuring "overfat" and healthy weight than the old height/weight charts, it's still a fairly crude estimator, and is insensitive to individual differences in body fat and muscle. Even with a BMI of 25, 26, or 27, you may not be overfat if you've been working out and much of your weight comes from muscle.

How to Find Out Your BMI

To use this chart, find your height on the left column and move your finger over to the weight that's closest to your own. For instance, if you're 5 feet 5 inches tall (5'5" in the chart) and 153 pounds, your Body Mass Index (BMI) is close to 25. Researchers generally find that starting at a BMI of 25, the higher your BMI, the greater your risk for heart disease. That risk is just a little higher between 25 and 27 than it is under 25. After a BMI of 27, risk steadily increases.

Height (feet/inches)	BMI 25 Low Risk	BMI 27 Increased Risk	BMI 30 High Risk
	Body Weight		
4'8"	119	129	143
4'9"	124	133	148
5'0"	128	138	153
5'1"	132	143	158
5'2"	136	147	164
5'3"	141	152	169
5'4"	145	157	174
5'5"	150	162	180
5'6"	155	167	186
5'7"	159	172	191
5'8"	164	177	197
5'9"	169	182	203
5'10"	174	188	207
5'11"	179	193	215
6'0"	184	199	221
6'1"	189	204	227
6'2"	194	210	233
6'3"	200	216	240
6'4"	205	221	246

(Source: Adapted with permission: W/H —George A. Bray, M.D., copyright, 1988)

Waist Size and Risk

Another way to assess your risk of heart disease is to get out a tape measure and measure the widest part of your belly. High risk for women is anything over 35 inches; for men, more than 40 inches.

Ten Bottom-Line Diet Tips
to Keep the Cardiologist Away

1. The number one piece of advice to keep heart disease away has to be: eat more fatty fish, high in omega-3 fatty acids—at least an ounce a day or a fish serving two or three times a week.
2. Also, go heavy on garlic, onions, and all kinds of other vegetables and fruits to keep plenty of antioxidants in the blood, as well as anticoagulants that protect arteries from clogging.
3. Take in 25 to 30 grams of fiber daily, including soluble fiber found in oats, psyllium, beans, and vegetables.
4. Eat magnesium-rich foods such as beans, greens, and wheat bran.
5. Eat foods rich in folic acid (greens, orange juice), B6 (fortified cereal, beans), and B12 (shellfish, low-fat dairy, lean meats).
6. Shun fatty animal foods, such as high-fat meat and high-fat dairy products.
7. Use olive oil and canola oil.

8. If you drink alcohol, a drink or two a day, especially of red wine with meals, may act as antidotes to heart disease; but if you do not already use alcohol, do not start drinking, because the dangers can well outweigh the benefits. If you drink more than two drinks a day, cut down. Heavy drinking harms your heart and your general health and boosts chances of death.

9. Restrict coffee to a couple of cups a day if you have heartbeat irregularities. There is no known advantage in switching to decaf to prevent heart disease.

10. If you're overweight, lose weight gradually by eating a balanced diet and increasing exercise.

Chapter 2

The Ultimate Anticholesterol Diet

Foods That Can Help Control Cholesterol:
Beans • Soy • Oats • Apples • Carrots • Olive Oil • Avocados • Almonds • Walnuts • Garlic • Onions • Seafood, Especially Fatty Fish • Fruits and Vegetables Rich in Vitamin C and Beta Carotene • Tea • Foods High in Soluble Fiber • Calcium-Rich Foods • Moderate Alcohol
Foods That Can Increase Harmful Cholesterol:
Foods High in Saturated Fat, Trans Fat, and Cholesterol

Cholesterol—that yellow, waxy, fatty stuff—in your blood is one reason your arteries become depositories for biological muck called plaque that narrows the blood vessels and shortens the gap between you and heart disease. Yet, cholesterol is not a simple matter. Some components of cholesterol are dangerous to arteries, while others are beneficial. Furthermore, what you eat may actually detoxify detrimental cholesterol so it cannot harm arteries. Regardless of cholesterol's complexities, one thing is undeniable: What you eat can put a striking dent in dangerous cholesterol, and more spectacularly, according to new findings, change its character so it is not so deadly!

This radical new way of controlling cholesterol by detoxifying it, according to new research, promises to dramatically slow the progression of atherosclerosis by 50 to 70 percent and even help reverse existing artery clogging by shrinking the clumps of plaque on artery walls, says leading researcher Daniel Steinberg, M.D., at the University of California School of Medicine in San Diego. "We can now attack the disease at the artery wall as well as by simply lowering cholesterol. It's very exciting," he says.

How You Can Use Food to Control Cholesterol

Essentially, you should eat in a way to lower one type of cholesterol, called LDL (low-density lipoprotein), and boost another type, known as HDL (high-density lipoprotein). That's because the LDLs are "bad guys" that serve as raw material to clog arteries. In contrast, the good guy HDLs gobble up the LDL "villains" and cart them to the liver, where they are annihilated. Generally, the more HDL and the less LDL you have in your blood, the safer your arteries. Certain foods help bring this about by preventing or destroying detrimental LDLs and creating beneficial HDLs.

Because of new knowledge about how cholesterol

causes artery damage, it's now possible to control cholesterol with food in ways unimagined even several years ago. A theory originally proposed by Dr. Steinberg and colleagues, now widely accepted, explains how arteries get clogged: Special forms of oxygen known as free radicals in the blood collide with fatty LDL cholesterol molecules, oxidizing them. The LDL then turns rancid, much as unrefrigerated butter does. In this altered form it is quickly gobbled up by cells called macrophages. Stuffed with fat globules, the macrophages enlarge into dreaded "foam cells," which insinuate themselves into artery walls, triggering artery destruction. If you can prevent this toxic transformation, your LDL cholesterol may remain relatively harmless. So the issue is not just how much LDL cholesterol your blood contains, but how much of it is "toxic oxidized LDL," capable of clogging your arteries. Most heart authorities now believe that LDL cholesterol is not so dangerous to arteries unless it is converted into a toxic form by oxygen free radicals in your blood.

That's where diet can be a powerful weapon. Extensive evidence shows you can block LDL's toxic transformation, and thus its awesome hazards, by eating foods packed with protective antioxidants. This means you might intervene at the very *genesis of atherosclerosis* at every stage of life, blocking the cascade of arterial events that create clogged arteries, heart attacks, and strokes. It is a thrilling prospect with substantial evidence to back it up.

- **BOTTOM LINE:** To combat hazardous blood cholesterol, you can reduce bad LDL cholesterol, boost good HDL cholesterol, and keep as much as possible of your LDL from becoming toxic to your arteries. Here are your best bets for doing it with diet.

Magic Beans

Eat dried beans or legumes. They are one of nature's cheapest, most widely available, fastest-acting, and safest cholesterol-fighting drugs. They consistently strike down cholesterol, studies show. According to James Anderson, M.D., of the University of Kentucky College of Medicine, eating a cup of cooked dried beans a day generally suppresses bad cholesterol about 20 percent. You can expect results in three weeks or so. All types of beans work—pintos, black, navy, kidney, lentils, chickpeas, soybeans—even plain old canned baked beans. In one test a half cup of Campbell's canned baked beans depressed cholesterol 12 percent in middle-aged men with high cholesterol who ate a typical high-fat American diet.

A cup of beans a day also drives up good HDLs about 9 percent, not immediately, but usually after a year or two. And beans improve the critical HDL/LDL cholesterol ratio by 17 percent, according to one test. Dr. Anderson's advice: For best results, spread the beans out during the day; for example, eat a half cup at lunch, another half cup at night. Beans contain at least six cholesterol-cutting compounds;

the main one may be soluble fiber.

The Gas Problem: No question, beans can cause gas. Soaking and rinsing beans several times can remove some of the gas-producing sugars, say U.S. Department of Agriculture researchers. Always discard the soaking water and add fresh water for cooking. New commercial anti-gas products found in your supermarket, such as Beano and BeSure, can help. Adding garlic and ginger to a pot of beans can also reduce beans' gas-producing properties, according to research in India.

"Most people can lower cholesterol by eating two-thirds of a cup of oat bran cereal or one cup of beans per day."

—James Anderson, M.D.,
University of Kentucky School of Medicine

How to Buy and Prepare Beans

At the Market: If you have time to cook them, buy uncooked dried beans. Among canned beans, the best choice is vegetarian low-fat style. Canned baked beans in tomato sauce have about 4 percent of calories from fat. That's compared to 20 to 30 percent fat calories in canned pork and beans and 40 percent in canned franks and beans and refried beans. Be aware that canned beans pack excess sodium—typically 400 to 600 milligrams in a half cup. Drain and rinse canned beans to wash away the sodium in the canning liquid.

In the Kitchen: You can store dried beans in a cool place in well-sealed containers for up to one year. After they are cooked, they keep in the refrigerator a few days. Generally, most dried beans are presoaked; if not, extend the cooking time an hour or so. You should use about two cups of water for every one-half cup of presoaked dried beans, and cook for about an hour. Exceptions: lentils and split peas do not need presoaking; they take only a cup and a half of water and cook in twenty to thirty-five minutes. Soybeans need about two and a half hours to cook.

Legumes double or triple in size during cooking. One-half cup dry beans (about three and a half ounces) equals about one and a half cups cooked. Skim off scum that rises to the surface.

Quick Soak: You can let dried beans soak overnight before cooking, but it's really not necessary except for soybeans. Usually boiling dried beans for a couple of minutes and letting them soak for an hour before cooking does the trick. Even faster: Boil beans over medium heat for ten minutes. Let them soak, covered, for thirty minutes before cooking.

Super Soy— Government-Approved

Soy, particularly soy protein, is such a potent cholesterol reducer that it even got the Food and Drug Administration's (FDA) approval. The FDA recently passed a ruling that the food labels on certain soy foods can make the claim that soy protein lowers the risk of heart disease. This is a big deal; the FDA has allowed only a handful of health claims.

The FDA's review of the research concluded that 25 grams of soy protein per day have a cholesterol-lowering effect. More may work even better. A review of thirty-eight human studies in a *New England Journal of Medicine* article by University of Kentucky's James Anderson, M.D., found that eating an average 47 grams (about 1.6 ounces) of soy protein daily in place of animal protein depressed bad LDL cholesterol 13 percent, triglycerides 10 percent, and raised good HDL cholesterol 2.5 percent.

That's a lot of soy—more than a quart of soy milk a day—but eating less lowers cholesterol to a lesser degree, says Dr. Anderson. Further, the more soy foods you eat and the higher your cholesterol, the greater the impact on cholesterol. Dr. Anderson concluded that eating soy protein regularly could potentially reduce heart disease risk 25 to 30 percent.

The secret seems to be the soy protein, found in such foods as whole and split soybeans, soy milk, tofu, textured soy protein and tempeh, and foods made with soy flour, but not in soy sauce and soybean oil. Researchers suspect that it's something about the amino acids (protein building blocks) in soy foods that lower cholesterol. Soy's amino acid content is different from animal and most other vegetable proteins, and appears to alter the way cholesterol is made and used in the liver.

Soybeans also possess a unique chemical called genistein, a plant hormone that helps lower blood cholesterol, says researcher Stephen Barnes at the University of Alabama at Birmingham. You get genistein in soy protein foods such as tofu, soy milk, soy flour, textured soy protein, and soybeans themselves. Soy sauce, soybean oil, and soy-based ice cream are *not* sources of genistein.

Oat Power

Eat oats to drive down cholesterol. Dutch scientists discovered the anticholesterol power of oats three decades ago, and it's now been confirmed by dozens of studies, says Michael C. Davidson, M.D., assistant professor of cardiology at Rush-Presbyterian-St. Luke's Medical Center in Chicago. It does not take fantastic amounts. "A medium-sized bowl of cooked oat bran or a large bowl of oatmeal did the job," Dr. Davidson reported in a recent study. Indeed, he concluded that the biggest dose you ever need to eat is two ounces of oat bran a day, or two-thirds of a cup dry. That amount reduced detrimental cholesterol 16 percent in those eating a low-fat diet. Half that much—an ounce or a third of a cup dry—cut cholesterol 10 percent. However, shoveling in three daily ounces of oat bran *did not lower cholesterol further*.

Oatmeal worked, too, but it takes twice as much oatmeal as oat bran for the same impact. Most telling, says Dr. Davidson, was the fact that oats lowered cholesterol enough to save one-third of the group from potent cholesterol-lowering drugs. Even a couple of ounces of instant oats a day depressed high blood cholesterol by 6 percent after two months, according to another study.

You can also expect a big bowl of oat bran daily to boost good HDL cholesterol about 15 percent after two or three months, says Dr. Davidson.

Oats' main cholesterol-busting substance is beta glucans, a soluble gummy fiber that jells in the intestinal tract. This interferes with the absorption and production of cholesterol, so more of it is removed from the bloodstream.

Oat Bran Mysteries: What You Need to Know

Oats work better on some people than on others. Some studies find large cholesterol drops of up to 20 percent, others, a modest 3 or 4 percent. One widely publicized Harvard study declared that oats had zero effect. Here are possible reasons for the variations in research findings:

- Commercial oat brans vary widely in their content of soluble fiber, namely beta glucans, and thus in pharmacological power. Tests show typical soluble fiber percentages in oat brans range from 8 to 28 percent. But some have little or no beta glucans—the main active agent, says Gene Spiller, Ph.D., a noted fiber researcher and director of the Health Research and Studies Center in California. Thus, they don't work. His advice: If "soluble fiber" content is noted on the label, choose an oat bran with the most. Or stick with oatmeal; it always contains some beta glucans, he says.
- Oat bran, like any pharmacological agent, affects individuals differently. Wendy Demark-Wahnefried,

Ph.D., now at Duke University, found that men and women eating 1.7 ounces of cooked oat bran, or 1.5 ounces of Quaker's cold oat-bran cereal daily, had average dips in cholesterol of 10 to 17 percent. Still, 33 percent of the oat bran eaters and 27 percent on low-fat diets had no cholesterol drops at all. In contrast, cholesterol fell an astonishing 80 to 100 points in others. The message, says Dr. Demark-Wahnefried, is that oats, like other natural or man-made drugs, are not a universal panacea. But if it works for you, it can make a tremendous difference. The only way to find out is to try it.

- If your cholesterol is high—above 230—the more apt oats are to bring it down. (The same applies to beans and other high-soluble-fiber foods.) Oats do not cut cholesterol substantially if it is already normal or fairly low—"in those who don't need it," says Dr. Anderson. Also, oats depress cholesterol even in those eating a typical American high-fat diet. In one study, two ounces daily of oat bran reduced bad LDL cholesterol 8.5 percent in men with high cholesterol (210 to 325) who ate an extravagant 41 percent of calories from fat.

- Oat power may vary with age and gender. Young women sometimes get virtually no cholesterol reduction from oats, while older women often have "a marked drop in cholesterol," concluded a recent review. Men of all ages seem to get intermediate effects.

- **BOTTOM LINE:** If your cholesterol is high—over 230—a daily bowl of oat bran is likely to lower it. If it is already low, oats will probably do zilch. Also, you can't expect additional benefits from eating more than two-thirds of a cup of dry oat bran or one and one-third cups of dry oatmeal a day, according to a review of the evidence by Cynthia M. Ripsin of the University of Minnesota.

A Garlic Clove a Day

Eat garlic if you are concerned about cholesterol. About twenty published human tests show that fresh garlic and some garlic preparations reduce cholesterol. Research indicates that three fresh garlic cloves a day may lower cholesterol an average 10 percent and up to 15 percent in some people. (Of course, less may work to a lesser degree.) Fully six compounds in garlic have been identified that lower cholesterol by suppressing the liver's synthesis of cholesterol. However, it is thought that allicin is the primary cholesterol-lowering compound in garlic, according to Larry Lawson, Ph.D., author of a recent textbook on garlic. Allicin is released when garlic is crushed or cooked lightly.

"The humble garlic clove is increasingly being shown to have exciting potential as a safe prophylactic for everyday use against cardiovascular risk factors."
—British physician J. Grunwald

In one controlled test, at L.T.M. Medical College in Bombay, fifty subjects who ate three raw garlic cloves every morning for two months saw their cholesterol drop about 15 percent—down from an average 213 to 180. Their blood-clotting factors also improved dramatically. In another study, at Bastyr College in Seattle, a daily dose of garlic oil from three fresh garlic cloves drove cholesterol down 7 percent in a month, but more important, raised good type HDL 23 percent!

Contradictory Research: In 1998 a German study made headlines, casting doubt on garlic's ability to lower cholesterol. In the study, people with high blood cholesterol took either an odorless powdered garlic tablet (the equivalent of about a clove of fresh garlic) or a placebo (dummy pill) for twelve weeks. At the trial's end, neither group lowered blood cholesterol, and the researchers concluded that the garlic powder was ineffective. However, experts point out this one study is pitted against many others that consistently show that garlic *does* lower cholesterol.

Note: Fresh garlic cooked or raw, garlic powder, and garlic salt all contain the presumed cholesterol-lowering agents. More than three raw cloves daily can cause diarrhea and stomach upset.

Half an Onion a Day

Raw onion is one of the few foods that boost beneficial HDL cholesterol, according to Victor Gurewich, a cardiologist and professor of medicine at Harvard Medical School. He reported that half a raw onion, or the equivalent in juice, raised HDLs an average 30 percent in most people with heart disease or cholesterol problems. Dr. Gurewich got the onion tip from folklore medicine and started testing it in his clinic. It was so successful, he advises all his patients to eat onions. The more you cook the onions, however, the more they lose their HDL-raising powers. (Cooked onions fight heart disease in other ways.) Dr. Gurewich does not know which chemicals in onions boost HDLs. He says it could be one or more of hundreds. The onion therapy works in about 70 percent of patients. If you can't eat half a raw onion a day, eat less. Any amount may help lift all-important HDLs.

High on Salmon

To boost beneficial HDLs, eat fatty fish, like salmon and mackerel, full of omega-3 fatty acids. They can hike HDLs, even if they are already normal. In a test,

Spice Attack!

Use lots of sage, rosemary, thyme, and cumin. These seasonings have been shown to prevent toxic chemical changes in LDL cholesterol that enable it to clog arteries. The active cholesterol-fighting agents in herbs and spices: antioxidants.

men with normal cholesterol feasted on salmon entrees for lunch and dinner for about forty days. Their HDLs shot up. Most important, according to study director Gary J. Nelson, Ph.D., of the U.S. Department of Agriculture's Western Human Nutrition Research Center in San Francisco, one particular lifesaving fraction of HDL jumped an average 10 percent. He says this specific HDL fraction is closely linked to thwarting heart disease. Moreover, the HDL hike came within twenty days! The results were surprisingly rapid, says Dr. Nelson, indicating a quick cholesterol and heart dividend from eating fatty fish.

How much salmon? The men ate "the maximum dose"—about a pound of fresh salmon a day. High doses are standard for research purposes to detect an effect. But less would also boost HDLs to a lesser degree, says Dr. Nelson. Moreover, if your HDLs are subnormal, you can expect even higher rises from eating fish. Since the active agent is thought to be omega-3 fatty acids, other oil-rich fish (mackerel, herring, sardines, tuna) would similarly drive up HDLs.

The salmon also depressed triglycerides, as eating fatty fish usually does.

Olive Oil Does It All

It's hard to rave enough about the bountiful benefits of olive oil to arteries and cholesterol. It is a triple savior. Olive oil both cuts bad LDL cholesterol and slightly raises or keeps good HDL the same, improving your heart-saving HDL/LDL ratio. In contrast, oils such as corn, soybean, safflower, and sunflower lower both good HDL and detrimental LDL. A major study even declared olive oil superior to the standard recommended low-fat diet in combating cholesterol. When subjects ate 41 percent of their calories in fat, most of it from olive oil, their bad LDL cholesterol sank more than when they ate a diet with half as much fat. Additionally, good HDLs rose on the olive oil diet and sank on the low-fat diet.

The clincher is that olive oil also helps defuse bad type cholesterol, rendering it less capable of destroying arteries. Studies by the University of California's Dr. Daniel Steinberg, as well as by researchers in Israel, find that olive oil dramatically thwarts toxic oxidation of LDL cholesterol. In a landmark study, Dr. Steinberg and colleagues gave one group of healthy volunteers about 40 percent of their calories in monounsaturated fat, equal to about three tablespoons of olive oil a day. Others ate regular safflower oil low in monounsaturated fatty acids. Then researchers examined the bad type LDL cholesterol from both groups. Remarkably, the

LDL of the monounsaturated oil eaters *was only half as likely to become oxidized and thus able to clog arteries!* This does not mean you should swill down olive oil. But it does suggest that when you eat fat, the olive oil monounsaturated type is a good choice to forestall artery clogging.

"From many surveys on the island of Crete, I have the impression that centenarians are common among farmers, whose breakfast is often only a wine glass of olive oil."
—Dr. Ancel Keys, renowned epidemiologist

Raves for Almonds and Walnuts

How could nuts be good for cholesterol? Aren't they high in fat? Yes, but 50 to 80 percent of the fat in nuts is monounsaturated, known to depress cholesterol and discourage LDL from oxidizing. Dr. Gene Spiller of the Health Research and Studies Center in Los Altos, California, had men and women with fairly high cholesterol, averaging around 251, eat three and a half ounces of almonds a day for four weeks. Others ate equal amounts of fat from cheese or olive oil.

The average cholesterol of the almond eaters sank by 12 percent, the olive oil group dropped by 4 percent, and the cheese group (no surprise!) went up 5 percent. Even more impressive was the plunge in artery-clogging LDL cholesterol: down 16 percent in almond eaters, 5 percent in the olive oil group, and up 6 percent in cheese eaters. It makes sense that the almonds and olive oil were both beneficial, says Dr. Spiller, because most of the fat in these foods is chemically identical. Thus, if olive oil is good for the heart, as much research shows, so is almond oil.

Walnuts work, too, according to research by Dr. Joan Sabate of Loma Linda University. He studied subjects with normal blood cholesterol. All were on a low-fat diet. But for one month they ate 20 percent of their calories in walnuts (about two ounces of walnuts in a daily 1,800 calorie diet). For another month, they ate no nuts. On the no-nuts diet, their cholesterol dropped an average 6 percent. But on the walnut-eating regimen, their cholesterol fell 18 percent! Average cholesterol dropped 22 points. Thus, walnuts added a cholesterol-reducing wallop even to an ordinary low-fat diet. As Dr. William Castelli of the Framingham Heart Study observed, "It looks like folks on nuts will do better than everyone else."

Nuts are a prominent part of the so-called Mediterranean diet that some Harvard researchers favor over the American low-fat (less than 30 percent fat calories) diet. A recent study found that following a Mediterranean diet (low in meat and high in fruits, vegetables, legumes, grains, cereals, and monounsaturated fats) after a heart attack was 70 percent more lifesaving than eating a low-fat diet. Nuts have other nutrient advantages besides good fat: they're high in magnesium, potassium, folic acid, and calcium, and are one of the few good dietary sources of vitamin E.

Both Drs. Spiller and Sabate, however, caution you

not to eat so many nuts you gain weight. (Nuts have about 170 calories per ounce, and dry roasted nuts are not significantly lower in calories and fat than oil-roasted nuts.) The point is to eat a few nuts a day as a substitute for other sources of fat and calories. "It's an easy way to improve cholesterol," says Dr. Sabate.

Avocados, Yes!

It's surprising but true that eating avocados can decidedly lower your cholesterol. Avocados have rich concentrations of the same type of cholesterol-improving monounsaturated fat as almonds and olive oil. Israeli investigators found that three months of eating avocados, as well as almonds and olive oil, cut detrimental LDL cholesterol about 12 percent in a group of men. Australian cardiologists at the Wesley Medical Centre in Queensland recently found that eating avocados (one-half to one and a half avocados a day) beat out a low-fat diet in reducing cholesterol. In their test, fifteen women ate a high-carbohydrate diet, a low-fat diet (20 percent fat calories), and an avocado high-fat diet (37 percent fat calories), each for three weeks. The raw avocados were put in salads or spread on bread or crackers.

The results: average cholesterol dipped 4.9 percent on the low-fat diet compared with nearly twice as much—8.2 percent—on the avocado diet. Most alarming, the low-fat diet wiped out good HDL cholesterol, lowering it a whopping 14 percent, but did not lower bad LDL cholesterol. Very low fat diets often do this. In contrast, the avocados attacked only detrimental LDLs. Investigators noted that avocados also protected arteries against oxidative damage that makes cholesterol dangerous.

Extrapolating from this research, investigators estimate that if heart patients included avocados in their diet, their risk of future heart attacks would drop 10 to 20 percent, and death rates 4 to 8 percent, in three to five years.

Avocado Profile

One ounce (two tablespoons) of a typical California (Haas) avocado contains 52 calories, 4.8 grams of fat (73 percent monounsaturated, 17 percent saturated), 30 IU vitamin A, 0.9 IU vitamin E, 24 micrograms folic acid, 2 mg sodium, 158 mg potassium. Like other fruits, avocado is free of cholesterol.

Ways to Eat Heart-Saving Avocados

• Add avocado slices or mashed avocado to sandwiches, such as turkey, ham, chicken, or tuna salad. Or spread sandwich bread with mashed avocado.

- Sprinkle a little lemon juice and salt on half an unpeeled avocado and eat it with a spoon as they do in Latin America.
- Fill an avocado half with seafood, poultry, rice, or vegetable salads.
- Add avocado slices, chunks, or cubes at the last minute to salads. For a simple salad, mix slices of avocados and onions with olive oil and vinegar.
- Use avocado instead of cheese in a chef's salad. The substitution slashes fat grams in half and saturated fat by almost 90 percent.
- Spread mashed avocado on bread, toast, bagels, English muffins. Compare: one tablespoon of avocado contains 2.5 grams of fat; mayonnaise, 11 grams; butter, 12 grams.
- Garnish chilled soups with avocado slices or cubes.
- Add diced avocado to salsas.

Caution: Eating large amounts of avocados can interact with the blood-thinning drug Coumadin, promoting bleeding, according to Canadian researchers.

- **BOTTOM LINE:** Although olive oil, almonds, and avocados are high in fat, most of it is monounsaturated fat that tends to improve cholesterol and dramatically protect rather than destroy arteries.

Cure Your Cholesterol With Strawberries

Give your blood an injection of vitamin C, vitamin E, and other antioxidants by eating fruits and vegetables. They are anticholesterol superfoods. Vitamin C combats cholesterol dangers two important ways. It acts as a bodyguard for HDLs that constantly cleanse your arteries of the bad stuff. And both vitamins C and E are potent at blocking transformation of LDL cholesterol that destroys arteries. For example, men and women who ate 180 milligrams of vitamin C a day (the amount in a cup of strawberries plus a cup of broccoli) had 11 percent higher HDLs than those who ate one-third as much vitamin C, according to Dr. Judith Hallfrisch of the U.S. Department of Agriculture. Women getting the vitamin C in just three oranges had the very highest artery-protecting HDL cholesterol. One theory is that vitamin C protects HDLs from attack and destruction by rampaging oxygen free radicals.

And you have only to consider the arteries of experimental monkeys to understand how vital vitamin C and E are to preventing artery clogging. Anthony J. Verlangieri, Ph.D., at the University of Mississippi's Atherosclerosis Research Laboratory, studied monkeys for six years. When he fed them lard and cholesterol and very little vitamin C and E, their arteries became severely damaged and clogged. But he was able to block the arterial deterioration and even reverse it by adding vitamin C and E to the high-fat diet. For example, fat-fed monkeys that got vitamin E had only one-third the artery blockage. More startling, feeding the monkeys relatively low doses of the vitamins for a couple of years actually reversed the arterial blockage by 8 to 33 percent!

The antioxidant vitamins work, say experts, by zapping oxygen free radicals that otherwise would turn LDL cholesterol toxic and dangerous. It doesn't take much to mount this defense, says Harvard researcher Balz Frei, Ph.D. He says eating a mere 160 milligrams of vitamin C a day—a couple of large oranges—gives body tissues enough ammunition to block free radicals and cripple LDL's ability to infiltrate arteries. The National Cancer Institute recommendation of at least five fruits and vegetables a day easily adds up to 200 to 300 mg of vitamin C. (For foods rich in vitamins C and E, see Appendix, pages 291–92 and 293–94.)

Smokers Alert! If you smoke, you need at least twice as much vitamin C as nonsmokers, because your body uses up gobs of vitamin C trying to combat free radicals in smoke. Smokers consistently have low blood levels of vitamin C. So do "passive smokers," who inhale secondhand smoke.

Cooking With Vitamin C

At the Grocery: Head for the produce counter. Vitamin C super foods are fruits and vegetables, specifically red and green sweet bell peppers, cantaloupe, guava, papaya, kiwi fruit, strawberries, Brussels sprouts, grapefruit, oranges, tomatoes, broccoli, cauliflower. Frozen fruits and vegetables retain vitamin C; canned ones have less. However, a good bet are canned pimentos or roasted red peppers to put in antipastos, on bread, or used alone as a salad with olive oil and garlic—four ounces deliver 105 milligrams of vitamin C, 50 percent more than an orange. Shy away from processed artificial fruit drinks, high in water and added vitamin C, but low in juice. They are not a health bargain. Note: red bell peppers have 50 percent more vitamin C than green bell peppers.

At Home: Vitamin C is unstable, thus diminished by cooking and storing. Cook vegetables only until tender. Microwaving and stir-frying are best to preserve vitamin C. USDA tests found that cooking a vegetable, such as broccoli, in half a cup of water destroyed 50 percent of the vitamin C—the same as using four cups of water. Microwaving destroyed only 15 percent. Refrigerated raw vegetables can lose one-third of their vitamin C in a few days; and cooked refrigerated vegetables, one-half to two-thirds of their C after two or three days. Best guarantee of getting all the vitamin C a vegetable has to offer: eat it raw or lightly cooked, soon after buying it.

Eating Out: It's easy to get vitamin C when eating out. The most reliable staple: orange or grapefruit juice. A small six-ounce glass has 60 to 80 milligrams. Fruit plates are another vitamin C powerhouse. At the breakfast bar or salad bar, grapefruit segments, mandarin oranges, strawberries, cantaloupe, kiwi, raw cauliflower, and broccoli are excellent vitamin C pick-ups. Tomato soup and tomato sauce on pasta are also good vitamin C sources. Always and anywhere, peeling and eating a whole orange is a sure way to get a vitamin C fix—about 70 milligrams. Overcooked vegetables, as on a cafeteria steam table, have lost much vitamin C.

Make Time for Tea

Among the many ways tea safeguards the heart is its effect on blood cholesterol. A study of 1,371 Japanese men over age 40, reported in the *British Medical Journal*, makes the case. Men who drank the most green tea had the lowest total blood cholesterol and triglycerides and best ratio of good HDL cholesterol to bad LDL cholesterol. Further, the amount of oxidized or dangerous type fats in the blood dropped, the more tea the men drank. In fact, heavy smokers who drank more than ten small-size Japanese cups of green tea daily had no more oxidized blood fats than nonsmokers. This suggests the tea neutralized harmful free radicals that promote clogging. Credit lies with naturally occurring antioxidant compounds in tea called flavonoids. In addition to tea, grapes, onions, apples, and wine are rich sources.

Two or three cups a day of green tea or black tea, with or without caffeine, should benefit cholesterol levels, say experts.

Take Two Apples, and . . .

Apples and other foods high in a soluble fiber called pectin can help drive down your cholesterol. French researchers had a group of middle-aged healthy men and women add two or three apples a day to their ordinary diet for a month. LDL cholesterol fell in 80 percent of them—and by more than 10 percent in half of them. Good HDL also went up. Interestingly, the apples had a greater impact on women. One woman's cholesterol plunged by 30 percent.

Similarly, David Gee, Ph.D., at Central Washington University, tested high-fiber apple slush left over from making apple juice. He had the apple fiber baked into cookies. When twenty-six men with fairly high cholesterol ate three apple cookies a day instead of a placebo cookie, their cholesterol dipped an average 7 percent. Each apple cookie had 15 grams of fiber—the amount in four or five apples, he says. Most experts mainly credit pectin in apples, the same stuff used in jelly to make it jell, with lowering cholesterol, although other apple components also play a part. As Dr. David Kritchevsky of the Wistar Institute in Philadelphia points out, a whole apple lowers cholesterol more than its pectin content predicts. "Something else is at work also," he says.

Carrots vs. Cholesterol

Count on carrots to help suppress bad cholesterol and raise good cholesterol. They, too, are full of anticholesterol soluble fiber, including pectin, say Philip Pfeffer, Ph.D., and Peter Hoagland, Ph.D., scientists at the U.S. Department of Agriculture's Eastern Regional Research Center. Dr. Pfeffer calculates that the fiber in a couple of carrots a day can lower cholesterol by 10 to 20 percent, which would bring many people with moderately high cholesterol into the normal range. After he started eating a couple of carrots a day, his own blood cholesterol dived around 20 percent.

A Canadian test found that men who ate about two and a half raw carrots every day saw their cholesterol sink an average 11 percent. According to a German study, the amount of beta carotene in one or two carrots also boosted good HDLs significantly. Drinking a cup and a quarter of carrot juice, containing 16 milligrams of beta carotene, reduced toxicity of bad type LDL cholesterol and its ability to clog arteries, according to Australian researchers.

The carrot fiber remains therapeutic whether the carrots are raw, cooked, frozen, canned, chopped, or liquefied, says Dr. Pfeffer.

Super Sources of Cholesterol-Fighting Fiber

Some authorities, such as James Anderson, M.D., insist that soluble fiber is the main cholesterol-lowering agent in foods, and that the more of such fiber in a food, the greater its powers to cut cholesterol. Here is Dr. Anderson's rundown of super sources of soluble fiber. He urges eating at least 6 grams of soluble fiber a day to fight bad cholesterol.

	Soluble Fiber Grams
Vegetables (1/2 cup)	
Brussels sprouts, cooked	2.0
Parsnips, cooked	1.8
Turnips, cooked	1.7
Okra, fresh	1.5
Peas, cooked	1.3
Broccoli, cooked	1.2
Onions, cooked	1.1
Carrots, cooked	1.1
Fruit	
Oranges, flesh only (1 small)	1.8
Apricots, fresh (4 medium)	1.8
Mangos, flesh only (1/2 small)	1.7
Cereal	
Oat bran, cooked (3/4 cup)	2.2
Oat bran cereal, cold (3/4 cup)	1.5
Oatmeal, uncooked (1/3 cup)	1.4

	Soluble Fiber Grams
Legumes, cooked (1/2 cup)	
Butter beans	2.7
Baked beans, canned	2.6
Black beans	2.4
Navy beans	2.2
White beans, canned	2.2
Kidney beans, canned	2.0
Chickpeas	1.3

Calcium-Rich Foods

Surprisingly, calcium may be a weapon against bad cholesterol. In a test by Margo A. Denke, of the University of Texas Southwestern Medical Center in Dallas, men with moderately high cholesterol ate a diet fairly high in beef and fat and low in calcium—410 milligrams daily. Then they switched to a high-calcium regimen of 2,200 milligrams per day. Their average total cholesterol dipped 6 percent. More important, their artery-clogging bad LDL cholesterol fell 11 percent.

Why the calcium worked is fascinating. It partly blocked absorption of saturated fat in the gastrointestinal tract. Such animal fats from meat, cheese, and butter are notorious at boosting cholesterol. If they are not absorbed, they can't raise cholesterol. Indeed, twice as much fat washed out in the men's stools during the high-calcium diets. You can't depend on calcium to cancel out the danger of a high-fat diet, but it may go a long way toward blunting its cholesterol-raising impact.

An easy way to get calcium is to consume low-fat or nonfat milk and yogurt. A glass of skim milk contains 300 milligrams, a cup of nonfat yogurt, up to 415 milligrams, depending on the brand. Still, some nondairy foods are also good sources. In Asian countries, vegetables and tofu often provide enough calcium. Indeed, studies show that you absorb more calcium from kale than from milk. However, you have to eat lots of kale to get as much calcium as you get in milk. (See Appendix, page 288, for a list of good calcium sources.)

What to Eat
to Lower Triglycerides

Another type of blood fat, triglycerides, may be more dangerous than previously thought. New evidence shows high levels can promote heart attacks, especially in women over age 50 and in men with poor LDL/HDL cholesterol ratios. Whereas the standard definition of normal triglycerides has been under 150 to 200, researchers at the University of Maryland Medical Center say a triglyceride level of more than 100 milligrams is too high and raises cardiac risk. A Finnish study found that men with bad cholesterol ratios and triglycerides over 203 mg/dL had almost quadruple the risk of heart attack. But if cholesterol ratios were okay, triglycerides were not a hazard. The problem is that low HDLs and high triglycerides usually go together.

Foods That Can Detoxify
Bad Cholesterol

Deliberately eat foods rich in antioxidants that may help keep your LDL cholesterol from becoming oxidized and toxic. So far scientists have zeroed in on five potent antioxidant protectors found in fruits, vegetables, grains, and nuts. Here are your best bets for defeating LDL's destructive transformation:

- Eat fruits and vegetables that are high in antioxidant vitamin C, beta carotene, and numerous flavonoid pigments.
- Eat oils, nuts, seeds, and grains, notably wheat germ, high in vitamin E.
- Eat foods high in antioxidant monounsaturated fatty acids, such as olive oil, almonds, and avocados, shown to reduce oxidation of LDLs.
- Restrict fats that are easily oxidized. Most easily oxidized are omega-6 vegetable fats such as corn, safflower, and sunflower seed oils.

Foods That Lower Triglycerides

The best dietary therapy is seafood. Studies consistently show that fish oil drives triglycerides down dramatically. In a study at Oregon Health Sciences University, a daily dose of fish oil—comparable to eating about seven ounces of salmon, mackerel, or sardines—slashed triglycerides more than 50 percent. Another test at the University of Washington had men eat shellfish instead of their usual protein (meat, eggs, milk, and cheese) twice a day for three weeks. Clams sent their triglycerides down 61 percent, oysters 51 percent, and crabs 23 percent.

Other good bets: A daily clove of garlic depressed triglycerides by about 13 percent in one study and by 25 percent in another. A half cup of dried beans depressed triglycerides 17 percent.

A low-fat diet can also lower triglycerides.

Foods That Can Raise Triglycerides

Refined sugar, refined flour, fruit juices, dried fruits, and excessive alcohol, especially from binge drinking. One or two drinks a day do not generally raise triglycerides, experts say.

Grape Lore Vindicated

Here's the newest addition to foods that can boost all-important HDL cholesterol. It's grape seed oil, a mild salad oil squeezed from the seeds of grapes, and sold in some specialty food stores. David T. Nash, a cardiologist at the State University of New York Health Science Center in Syracuse, tested grape seed oil on twenty-three men and women who had low HDLs—below 45. Every day for four weeks, they ate two tablespoons of grape seed oil in addition to their regular low-fat diet. Their HDLs went up an average 14 percent! "Some did not respond," says Dr. Nash, "but the HDLs did go up in more than half of them." Generally, those who already had the highest HDLs (above 55) were least likely to get further boosts from the grape seed oil.

A Nip, If You Drink, Improves Cholesterol

It's a well-established fact that a little beer, wine, or alcohol boosts beneficial HDLs. Typical is a British study showing that a glass or two of wine, beer, or a mixed drink daily boosted HDLs an average 7 percent. Another study found that 1.3 daily ounces of alcohol boosted HDLs by 17 percent. Even light drinking brings benefits. A study at the Oregon Health Sciences University found that women taking between four and thirty alcoholic drinks a month had higher HDLs than women drinking no more than four drinks a month.

Johns Hopkins investigators also found that men who drank a twelve-ounce domestic beer a day for two months pushed up blood levels of apolipoprotein A-1, which converts to HDLs. Researchers suggested that drinking a beer a day might well make the difference between health and heart attack.

It looks as if red wine is the best choice. Antioxidants in red grapes and red wine help prevent bad type LDL cholesterol from becoming oxidized and able to clog arteries, says Edwin Frankel at the University of California at Davis. He finds grape antioxidants as strong as vitamin E in such artery protection. In his tests, red wines contained ten times more antioxidants than white wines and blocked LDL oxidation by 46 to 100 percent compared with 3 to 6 percent for white wines.

Further, a couple of studies suggest that white wine may promote artery damage. Israeli researchers found that drinking white wine spurred a 34 percent increase in dangerous oxidation of LDL cholesterol in particular. In contrast, red wine depressed blood fat oxidation by 20 percent and LDL oxidation by 40 percent.

But beware of binge drinking. Downing seven to fourteen drinks a week all on Friday and Saturday night does not benefit cholesterol the same way spreading the alcohol out through the week does. Too much alcohol at one time can actually ruin HDL cholesterol and raise LDL, studies show.

- **BOTTOM LINE:** Although a little drinking may benefit cholesterol, most researchers oppose recommending drinking as a public health measure to fight heart disease, and stress that nobody, particularly people with a personal or family history of alcohol abuse, should take up drinking to try to improve cholesterol. And alcohol, even in moderation, may raise breast cancer risk, so those with a history of breast cancer should not take up drinking.

Shellfish Surprise

If you're afraid that eating shellfish will send your cholesterol sky-high, don't be. True, shellfish, especially shrimp, contains a moderate amount of cholesterol, but research consistently shows that cholesterol in food is not much of a threat. The real danger is fat, notably saturated fat that raises blood cholesterol and increases blood clotting. Shellfish is low in fat; for instance, shrimp contains only 1.2 grams of fat for four ounces, 10 percent of calories. Three ounces of a porterhouse steak has nearly 19 grams of fat, about 70 percent of calories, more than half of it harmful saturated fat. Most experts consider shrimp a good low-fat food; some research shows it can lower cholesterol when substituted for high-fat meats.

For instance, a new Harvard study finds that shrimp, as part of a low-fat diet, actually improves blood cholesterol, reducing heart disease risk. In the study, subjects on a low-fat diet ate about ten ounces of steamed shrimp daily, supplying 590 milligrams of cholesterol. Their bad LDL cholesterol did jump 7 percent, but that was offset by a 12 percent rise in good HDL cholesterol. Thus, the ratio of bad and good types cholesterol improved. Further triglycerides, another potentially dangerous blood fat, dropped 13 percent.

In tests by Marian Childs, Ph.D., a lipid expert formerly at the University of Washington, eighteen healthy men with normal cholesterol substituted specific shellfish for three-week periods for their ordinary animal-protein foods like meat and cheese.

Not a single one of six common shellfish (oysters, clams, crabs, mussels, shrimp, squid) boosted blood cholesterol. Just the opposite—the oyster, clam, and crab diets lowered both total cholesterol and detrimental LDL cholesterol. Oysters and mussels improved the good HDL cholesterol ratios.

All-around best for cholesterol, said Dr. Childs, were oysters, clams, and mussels. Crabs, too, were beneficial. Shrimp and squid did not raise cholesterol, but neither did they lower it. Thus, Dr. Childs does not recommend eating shrimp or squid to improve cholesterol.

Foods That Can Raise
Good HDL Cholesterol

- Olive oil
- Onions, raw
- Garlic
- Salmon, mackerel, sardines, tuna, and other fatty fish
- Oysters, mussels
- Grape seed oil
- Almonds
- Avocados
- Vitamin C–rich foods (bell peppers, broccoli, oranges)
- Beta carotene–rich foods (carrots, spinach, broccoli)
- Wine, beer, alcohol in moderation
- Tea

Caution: Very low fat diets (10 percent or less of calories from fat) depress HDLs.

Filter Out Coffee Threat

Coffee beans contain diterpenes, chemicals that can slightly raise blood cholesterol and triglycerides, recent research shows. Fortunately, these culprits are largely removed when coffee is brewed by the drip-filter method favored in the U.S. About 75 percent of all the coffee brewed in the United States is filtered. Instant coffee is also virtually free of the cholesterol-raising chemicals. Espresso contains moderate amounts. However, European style boiled coffee and Turkish style coffee contain high amounts of diterpenes and may boost cholesterol.

Dutch researchers solved the puzzle. They extracted a fatty substance, called a lipid factor, from European type boiled coffee. Volunteers who ate the "coffee lipid factor" did experience cholesterol rises of an average 23 percent—from 180 to 220—within six weeks, nearly all of it in detrimental LDLs. Apparently, the cholesterol-boosting chemical does not get into filtered coffee. Thus, it appears your cholesterol is safe from elevation by java if you stick to drip-made coffee. Interestingly, another study at Johns Hopkins University found that even if regular coffee did boost cholesterol slightly, it raised both good HDL and bad LDL equally, making no difference in heart disease risk.

So, if you drink coffee, make it the American way—by the drip method in which the brewed coffee goes through a filter, which traps the cholesterol-raising compounds.

Danger in Decaf?

Forget about switching to decaf to control cholesterol. For one thing, research does not condemn caffeine as a cholesterol-booster. In one Dutch test, forty-five men and women substituted five daily cups of decaf coffee for their five cups of regular coffee for six weeks.

The effect on their blood cholesterol was "essentially zero."

Further, there are increasing hints of hazard in decaf. Investigators at the University of California's Center for Progressive Atherosclerosis Management in Berkeley actually found that detrimental LDL cholesterol rose by roughly 6 percent in 181 healthy men with normal cholesterol when they switched from regular coffee to decaf. Apolipoprotein B, another heart disease risk factor, also went up.

However, cholesterol did not change in men who simply stopped drinking coffee, but did *not* switch to decaf. The Berkeley study's director, H. Robert Superko, calculates that switching to decaf might boost coronary artery disease risk about 10 percent. That's significant, he says, when you consider that 20 percent of the 139 billion cups of coffee Americans drink every year is decaf. Dr. Superko believes an unknown chemical in stronger robusta beans, commonly used to make decaf coffee, is at fault. Caffeinated coffee usually comes from weaker arabica beans.

The findings, surprising as they may seem, jibe with other recent studies, such as one at Harvard that detected a marginally higher heart disease risk in men drinking decaf coffee. The clear message: Don't depend on decaf to save you from high cholesterol.

Chocolate, Not Guilty

Will eating lots of chocolate raise your cholesterol? Theoretically, yes. But in actual fact, maybe not, according to tests at Pennsylvania State University. True, about 60 percent of the fat in chocolate is saturated. But it comes mainly from cocoa butter. And cocoa butter's main type of saturated fat is stearic acid, which, oddly, tests show does not elevate cholesterol, and may even lower it.

Penn State researchers checked it out. Investigators had young men with normal cholesterol (under 200) pig out on chocolate, cocoa butter, or plain old dairy butter for twenty-five days at a stretch. Thirty-one percent of their daily calories came from butterfat, chocolate, or cocoa butter. That meant ten ounces of pure chocolate a day. "It's like eating seven candy bars a day," said researcher Elaine McDonnell.

Still, the men's cholesterol did not rise significantly after eating either the chocolate or the cocoa butter. "Cocoa butter seems to be neutral as far as raising cholesterol," says McDonnell. In contrast, the men's average cholesterol (mostly detrimental LDL) soared 18 points during the butterfat binge.

Eggs and Cholesterol— The Real Story

How hazardous is eating foods such as eggs, liver, caviar, and some seafood—all bubbling over with cholesterol? The truth is that high-cholesterol foods are a minor cause of high blood cholesterol; saturated animal fat is the real enemy—fully four times more potent in boosting blood cholesterol levels. Early studies at Rockefeller University in New York revealed that a diet rich in cholesterol-laden eggs raised blood cholesterol in only two out of five people. That's because when you eat too much cholesterol, your liver automatically pumps less cholesterol into your bloodstream, so levels remain about the same or do not rise much.

A new comprehensive analysis of 224 scientific studies over twenty-five years by Wanda Howell, Ph.D., University of Arizona, concludes that eating cholesterol only slightly affects blood cholesterol. The primary villain is saturated animal fat, she says. Reducing food cholesterol probably won't do much good either, according to a British study showing that cutting out 50 milligrams of dietary cholesterol a day reduces blood cholesterol less than 1 point.

More remarkable, a 1999 large-scale Harvard study published in the *Journal of the American Medical Association* virtually exonerated eggs as a cause of heart disease. The analysis of nearly 120,000 men and women over a fourteen-year period found that eating as much as an egg a day did not raise the risk of coronary heart disease or stroke in healthy men or women. Indeed, the researchers concluded that eating eggs might benefit good HDL cholesterol and triglycerides, possibly by supplying antioxidants and other nutrients that outweighed any small rise in detrimental blood cholesterol. One caution: the study did detect a higher heart disease risk in diabetics who ate more than one egg a day compared with less than one egg per week. The reason is unclear.

"Saturated fats are four times more likely to raise blood cholesterol levels than dietary cholesterol itself."

—John LaRosa, cardiologist,
George Washington University

Still, overdosing on cholesterol-rich foods is not a good idea either. Richard Shekelle, Ph.D., professor of epidemiology at the University of Texas Health Science Center in Houston, found that high-cholesterol eaters (700 milligrams a day or more—the amount in three egg yolks) had a shorter life span by an average three years.

It's also dangerous to fanatically avoid cholesterol-rich foods, according to Steven Zeisel at the University of North Carolina. You could develop a choline deficiency—choline is concentrated in high-cholesterol foods, particularly eggs. When Dr. Zeisel put healthy males on a choline-free diet for three weeks, they developed signs of liver dysfunction.

- **BOTTOM LINE:** Eat some cholesterol-rich foods to get sufficient choline, but don't overdo it. An egg a day is heart-safe for most people, says new Harvard research. Possible exception: people with diabetes.

The Most Dangerous Fats

Saturated Fat

Of all the things you can eat, the most likely to send cholesterol soaring is saturated animal type fat—the type concentrated in meat, poultry, and dairy products. That's been the word since cholesterol was first linked to diet, starting in the 1950s. Unquestionably, eating animal fat boosts bad LDL cholesterol in most people to varying degrees, and cutting out such fat usually lowers LDL cholesterol. That's why it's essential to shy away from butter, whole milk, cheese, beef, and pork fat and poultry skin to help keep your arteries from clogging.

Study after study shows the same thing: it is saturated type fat, not other monounsaturated or polyunsaturated fat, that boosts bad cholesterol. In one test, for example, subjects ate a high-fat diet—40 percent of calories from fat—except that one group ate the typical American diet high in saturated fat while the other group ate only 10 percent of calories in saturated fat. Almost immediately the blood cholesterol in the low-saturated-fat group dropped about 13 percent. Individuals vary greatly in their responses to saturated fats; a new study found that on average, LDL dropped about 1 percent for every 1 percent drop in saturated fat calories.

Cutting back on saturated fat is most likely to cause the biggest dips in those with fairly high cholesterol.

Results from the ongoing Harvard study of 80,000 women found that every 5 percent increase in calories from saturated fat, compared with the same amount of calories in the form of carbohydrates, increased risk from heart disease by 17 percent.

Trans Fat

Saturated fat isn't the only bad guy. Trans fatty acids, created when vegetable oils are hydrogenated or hardened into margarine or vegetable shortening, are proving to be as bad as saturated fats in raising cholesterol. The same Harvard study of 80,000 women that exposed the risk of saturated fat also found that those eating the highest level of trans fats (3 percent of total calories) increased their chances of getting heart disease by a third over the women eating the least trans fats (1 percent of calories). Looking at it another way, researchers concluded that adding a mere 2 percent of total calories from trans fatty acids nearly doubled odds of heart disease.

Some experts, including Harvard researcher Walter Willett, blame trans fatty acids, especially margarine, for high rates of heart disease. He notes that Americans' intake of trans fatty acids from hydrogenated vegetable fat zoomed from zero in 1900 to 5.5 percent of our total fat consumption in the 1960s. This unprecedented trans fatty acid binge closely paralleled our soaring rates of coronary heart disease. Dr. Willett once estimated that eating trans fats, particularly margarine, kills from 30,000 to 150,0000

Americans every year from heart disease.

Whenever you see these words on a food label ingredient list—"hydrogenated" or "partially hydrogenated" vegetable oil—especially as the first ingredient, it's a cause for alarm. It's another term for trans fatty acids. Look for labels that say "no trans fats," or do not list hydrogenated oils. However, some labels say "no trans" even though hydrogenated oil is listed as an ingredient. How is this possible? Because government regulations let companies list anything less than .5 gram of fat, including trans fat, as zero. If in doubt, you can simply subtract the grams of monounsaturated fat, polyunsaturated, and saturated fat from total fat grams. What's left is trans fat.

To be safe, restrict margarine, solid shortenings, and processed foods rich in hydrogenated or partially hydrogenated vegetable oils. If you use margarine, look for the brands that are trans-free, or choose soft (tub) or liquid margarine (lower in trans) over hard stick margarine. Packaged foods apt to be high in trans fats, according to the U.S. Department of Agriculture, are doughnuts, frozen French fries, pound cake, snack crackers, chocolate chip cookies, and microwave popcorn. Cutting out as little as 4 grams a day of trans fats could reduce your heart disease risk by half.

- **BOTTOM LINE:** You should get no more than 10 percent of your calories from saturated animal type fat, and less if possible. Drastically restrict your intake of trans fat by limiting foods with "partially hydrogenated vegetable oils" on the label.

Jack Sprat's Salvation

Can you eat meat and keep your cholesterol down? Yes, several studies suggest, if you trim off all possible cholesterol-raising fat. For example, researchers at Deakin University and the Royal Melbourne Hospital in Australia put a group of ten healthy men and women on a high-beef diet—about a pound of beef a day for three weeks. The beef was trimmed of all possible fat, making it so lean that the fat content was only 9 percent of calories. Rather than going up, their blood cholesterol dived an average 20 percent.

To clinch the case, the researchers added beef fat drippings during the fourth and fifth week of the experiment. The subjects' cholesterol shot up.

Fish Oil vs. a Strange Type of Cholesterol

If you have high levels of an odd type of cholesterol known as Lp(a)—pronounced "el pee little *a*"—you may be vulnerable to clogged arteries and heart attack at an early age, especially if your LDL cholesterol is also high. Some experts blame too much Lp(a) for a quarter of all heart attacks in people under age 60; they say that 10 to 25 percent of all Americans may have dangerously high Lp(a), which is genetically induced.

A traditional low-fat diet does not curb Lp(a). In fact, new research found that a diet low in fat and saturated fat actually *increased* Lp(a) levels. But there is hope: fish oil. Dr. Jorn Dyerberg, a leading Danish researcher, found that fish oil taken for nine months lowered abnormally high levels of Lp(a) by a remarkable 15 percent in a group of men. The daily dose: 4 grams—the equivalent of eating seven ounces of mackerel. A recent German study also found that high amounts of fish oil depressed Lp(a) an average 14 percent in thirty-five patients with coronary artery disease, although it was not beneficial in a few.

Simple tests are not yet available to widely detect elevated Lp(a). However, the threat provides one more rationale for eating fatty fish two or three times a week just in case you have high Lp(a). This mechanism may be one more mysterious way fish helps prevent heart attacks.

The Perils of Super-Low Fat

Unfortunately, you may think, as many people do, that the less fat you eat, the better for your cholesterol, arteries, and heart. But it's a dangerous myth and can put the hearts of healthy people in severe jeopardy, according to the latest research. There are several complex reasons why too little fat can seriously backfire and screw up your blood cholesterol, worsening your risk of cardiovascular disease.

Threat Number One: Going on a very low fat diet can actually increase levels of the most vicious form of LDL cholesterol, pushing you closer to a heart attack. New research reveals that not all LDL is equally harmful. So-called small dense LDL cholesterol particles are the worst villains. Larger LDL particles are more benign. In many people, switching to a low-fat diet spurs formation of dangerous small dense LDLs, and the more of these particles unleashed in your blood, the higher your heart disease odds. Generally, the greater the fat restriction, the graver the danger. In fact, this cruel joke is played on as many as two-thirds of normal healthy Americans who severely restrict fatty foods, says leading researcher Ronald Krauss, M.D., at the University of California in Berkeley. He explains that probably for genetic reasons, when some people restrict fat, great numbers of their large, safer LDL particles are replaced by the vicious small LDL particles. In a recent study, Dr. Krauss found that cutting fat calories from 46 percent to 24 percent caused increases of small LDL particles in about one-third of a group of healthy men and women. When fat restriction fell to 20 percent and below—about two-thirds of such normal healthy individuals suffered rises in small LDLs.

"Clearly, because of genetic differences a very low fat diet doesn't benefit everyone and can be harmful," says Dr. Krauss. Thus, encouraging a whole population to drastically restrict fat could backfire, he says.

On the other hand, if you already have lots of small dense LDLs, slashing certain fats, notably animal fat, can be lifesaving, says Dr. Krauss. Animal fat stimulates production of the dangerous small LDL particles; olive oil appears neutral, and fish oil reduces small LDLs. But how can you tell if high small LDL is a problem? Currently tests to measure levels of small LDL particles are not widely available outside research labs. But there are telltale signs: You probably have high small LDLs, says Dr. Krauss, if you have heart disease, high cholesterol, high blood pressure, high triglycerides along with low HDL cholesterol, diabetes, and/or are overweight.

Here's a warning sign that your low-fat diet is harmful: Your triglycerides go up and your good HDL cholesterol goes down.

Other ways to reduce the menacing small LDLs: exercise, weight loss, and pharmacological doses of niacin (1,500 milligrams a day) used only with a doctor's supervision.

Threat Number Two: A super low fat diet tends to drive down both your bad LDL cholesterol *and your good HDL cholesterol, leaving you as vulnerable to heart disease as before.* The reason: reducing fat often leads to a much higher intake of carbohydrates, which can have detrimental effects.

In recent tests, Dr. Gerald Reaven of Stanford University put healthy postmenopausal women on either a low-fat (25 percent of calories), high-carbohydrate diet (60 percent of calories) or a high-fat (45 percent), low-carbo (40 percent) diet. The fat was mostly monounsaturated, as in olive oil—not animal fat. On the low-fat, high-carbo diet, their triglycerides rose and good HDL dropped, dramatically boosting chances of developing heart disease, says Dr. Reaven. The high-carbo diet also drove up blood sugar and insulin levels, adding to heart disease risk. As women enter menopause, their risk of heart disease skyrockets; so this study indicates that the widely recommended solution—drastically cut fat and eat more carbohydrates—is a bad idea.

The same thing happened to men in research by Robert H. Knopp, University of Washington. To test the effect of an ultra low fat diet (such as that advocated by Dr. Dean Ornish), Dr. Knopp put 444 men with high cholesterol and/or high triglycerides on diets of 30 percent, 26 percent, 22 percent, and 18 percent fat calories for a year. The most beneficial fat intake was 30 percent for those with both high cholesterol and triglycerides, and 26 percent for those with only high cholesterol.

Slashing fat further did not additionally benefit cholesterol, blood pressure, blood sugar and insulin, or body weight. On the other hand, cutting fat to 22 or 18 percent made good HDL cholesterol go down and hazardous triglycerides go up, increasing chances of heart disease.

Harvard researcher Frank Sachs explains what's going on. You drastically cut fat in your diet, and your total cholesterol count drops from 260 to 210. But that is meaningless because your good HDL cholesterol also dives 20 percent, from 40 to 32. This means you are left with the same high *ratio* of total cholesterol to HDL of 6.5 as before—a ratio that still puts you at higher risk of heart attack than most Americans. The ratio is a far better predictor of heart disease than total cholesterol. Thus, Dr. Sacks says, after a stringent, demanding diet, you're no better off than before.

Threat Number Three: Strangely, a low-fat diet can *raise* levels of Lp(a), another hazardous type of blood cholesterol. That's what emerged from research led by Henry Ginsberg, M.D., of New York City's

Columbia University comparing two diets recommended by the American Heart Association. Their "Step 1" diet allows 30 percent or fewer calories from fat, no more than 10 percent saturated fat, and 300 milligrams of cholesterol. "Step 2" brings saturated fat down to 7 percent and cholesterol to 200 milligrams. When healthy adults were put on these diets, total and LDL cholesterol fell, as predicted; but researchers noticed to their surprise that Lp(a) went up. When people lowered their saturated fat intake from 15 percent to 6 percent of calories, Lp(a) rose by 15 percent. Ginsberg and his colleagues aren't sure whether the drop in LDL is worth the rise in Lp(a), citing the need for further research.

In contrast, eating monounsaturated fats like olive oil sinks bad LDLs but not protective HDLs. It makes more sense, says Dr. Sacks, to severely cut back on saturated animal fats, which decidedly boost bad LDL cholesterol, and to eat a higher-fat diet, rich in monounsaturated fats. He favors a Mediterranean type diet that provides 35 to 40 percent of calories from fat, with most of it coming from monounsaturated fats. If you go on a super low fat diet, have your HDLs checked within a few months to be sure you are actually helping, not harming, your cholesterol.

At a Harvard-sponsored conference, fifty worldwide experts went even further, concluding it doesn't matter how much total fat you eat, as long as you restrict animal fat and partially hydrogenated oils and eat an otherwise healthful diet of fruits, vegetables, legumes, whole grains, fish, nuts, and low-fat dairy products.

Bottom Line on Fat in the Diet

You may not benefit from a low-fat diet if:

- You replace fats with too many carbohydrates, mainly sugary "fat-free" foods.
- You cut too much good fat, such as olive oil and fish oil.
- Your genes react in ways to create bad "small dense" LDL cholesterol.

So, you should:

- Pay attention to the type of fat, not just total fat.
- Restrict saturated animal fat as much as possible; everyone agrees it's very dangerous.
- Avoid trans fatty acids, or partially hydrogenated fats, in margarines, crackers, doughnuts, and other processed foods. They appear as bad as or worse than animal fat.
- Substitute monounsaturated fat, olive oil, avocados, macadamia nut oil, and almonds for other fats. Such fat has been found potentially beneficial against stroke, disease, diabetes, and other chronic diseases.
- Use canola oil instead of corn, regular safflower, or soybean oils.
- Eat omega-3 fat in fatty fish, salmon, mackerel, sardines, herring, and walnuts.
- Eat a diet rich in plant foods—fruits, vegetables, beans, nuts, grains.

- Get your carbohydrates in fruits and vegetables, not in sugar or fat-free, high-sugar foods.
- Maintain normal weight by restricting overall calories and exercising.

Lose Some Weight

Losing weight, often just 10 pounds, pushes down your blood cholesterol and has an even more dramatic effect on blood triglycerides. A review of fourteen major studies found that losing 5 to 13 percent of your starting weight can lower cholesterol by up to 18 percent, and LDLs by even more. (But to keep the LDLs down, you should maintain that weight loss on a diet low in saturated fat.) Since every 1 percent reduction in blood cholesterol reduces your risk for heart disease by 2 percent, you can see how weight loss can dramatically decrease your heart disease risk. Even better, weight loss often leads to an increase in the good HDL cholesterol.

And research studies show that modest weight loss can knock down blood triglycerides as much as 44 percent. "However, most of you can expect high triglyceride levels to fall by 15 to 25 percent when you lose about 5 to 10 percent of your body weight," says Robert Eckel, M.D., professor of medicine at University of Colorado's Health Sciences Center and chairman of the American Heart Association's Nutrition Committee.

Can Cholesterol Ever Be Too Low?

Researchers are increasingly asking that question, and the unnerving answer may be yes. Very low levels of cholesterol—under 160—might be dangerous. In one major study of 350,000 middle-aged healthy men, Dr. James Neaton and colleagues of the University of Minnesota found that 6 percent had very low cholesterol levels and hardly a trace of heart disease. Twelve years later their death rate from heart attacks was half that of men with higher cholesterol counts of 200 to 239. However, the low-cholesterol men had other problems. They were twice as likely to have a bleeding stroke, to die of chronic obstructive lung disease, or commit suicide; they were three times as likely to have liver cancer, and five times as apt to die of alcoholism. Another worldwide study of 290,000 men and women, by Dr. David Jacobs at the University of Michigan, found that those with extra-low cholesterol had higher death rates from a variety of causes.

What's going on here? Nobody knows, but in recent years clues have emerged hinting that very low cholesterol may not be safe. Brain hemorrhages in which a weakened vessel "blows out," causing a hemorrhagic or bleeding stroke, appear to be a particular danger from super-low cholesterol, possibly because fragile membranes that cover brain cells need a minimum level of cholesterol to function properly. Interestingly, as average blood cholesterol levels rise among Japanese, their incredibly high rate of hemorrhagic stroke is declining. Low cholesterol has particularly been linked in studies to colon cancer and liver damage.

Then there is evidence that low cholesterol may somehow help induce depression, at least in elderly men. A study by Elizabeth L. Barrett-Connor, M.D., of the University of California at San Diego, found that such men with low cholesterol levels are strikingly more apt to suffer more symptoms of depression than their peers with moderate or high cholesterol. About 16 percent of the men 70 and older with low cholesterol of under 160 showed signs of mild to severe depression. Only 3 to 8 percent of the men with higher cholesterol were depressed.

Why? Dr. Barrett-Connor can only speculate that low cholesterol may somehow lessen concentrations of the brain chemical serotonin, leading to increased depression and aggression.

What is a safe minimum level? Researchers can only guess. It looks as if problems can start when total blood cholesterol dips below 160, some say.

> *"If I had a cholesterol level in the 160 to 190 range I would continue to do exactly what I was doing. I would not try to raise or lower it. But if I had a very low cholesterol level, like 120, I might actually consider trying to raise it."*
>
> —Dr. David Jacobs, epidemiologist,
> University of Michigan

Straight Talk About Diet Cures for Cholesterol

Diet therapy usually works best on those with the worst cholesterol—the highest LDLs or lowest HDLs—those who need help the most. It's probably futile and needless to try to use diet to push cholesterol lower if it is already normal or fairly low, under 180 to 200.

Also: Do not expect all foods to work the same way on all people. Individuals react differently, just as they do to cholesterol-lowering drugs. Experiment to find which foods work best for you. And do not rely on a single food or a few foods. Many different foods have cholesterol-fighting capabilities. Eat a variety of them. And remember, you do not need the super-high doses of each food found effective in studies. You can combine smaller portions of various foods to get similar cholesterol benefits.

Specifically:

- Eat plenty of fruits and vegetables, legumes, high-soluble fiber grains such as oats, and seafood, especially fatty fish like salmon, mackerel, sardines, and tuna.
- Cut back on saturated animal fats found in whole milk, cheese, meat fat, and poultry skin. This will help reduce your levels of detrimental LDL cholesterol and raise your good HDL cholesterol.
- Limit your intake of trans fatty acids found in hard margarines and many processed foods. This will help keep down LDL levels.
- Restrict omega-6 type vegetable oils, such as corn and safflower oil, also found in margarine, vegetable shortenings, and lots of processed foods. The oils are incorporated into LDL cholesterol particles where they are readily oxidized, converted to a toxic form that can destroy arteries.
- Don't go on an extremely low fat diet, it may be counterproductive. Eat a moderate amount of fat, favoring foods high in monounsaturated fats, such as olive oil and canola oil, avocados, and nuts.
- Extra-important: eat lots of antioxidant compounds concentrated in fruits, vegetables, nuts, and olive oil, including vitamin C, vitamin E, and beta carotene. They may keep LDL cholesterol safe from toxic changes that threaten arteries and promote heart attacks.
- Get enough calcium-rich foods, which may help reduce the absorption of saturated fat.
- Drink tea to help keep blood cholesterol in check.

- If you drink alcohol, a daily glass of wine, beer, or a drink of hard liquor may benefit HDL cholesterol. If you don't drink, do not take it up explicitly to try to improve cholesterol.
- Some other foods that studies show can help cut dangerous cholesterol are shiitake mushrooms, barley, rice bran, kelp (seaweed), skim milk, and green and black tea.

Chapter 3

Ten Foods That Fight Blood Clots

> Foods That May Discourage Blood Clots:
> Garlic • Onions • Hot Peppers • Black
> Mushrooms • Ginger and Cloves • Vegetables •
> Olive Oil • Seafood • Tea • Red Wine
> (Moderate Amounts)
> Foods That May Encourage Blood Clots: High-
> Fat Foods • Excessive Alcohol

Blood Clot Factors Can Save Your Life

The surprising fact is that the way your blood clots is probably the single greatest determinant of whether you suffer a heart attack, a stroke, or blood vessel damage. Experts now know that thrombotic factors—how the blood flows, its viscosity, its stickiness, the tendency for clots to form and enlarge—are primary in determining such catastrophes. And diet can have enormous influence on blood-clotting factors. Indeed, evidence suggests that the major influence of diet on heart disease has more to do with blood-clotting factors than with blood cholesterol. And the benefits of eating to modify blood clot factors are apt to kick in fairly quickly. A prominent French health official, Dr. Serge C. Renaud, says preventing blood clots can sharply cut your chances of heart attack within a year, whereas it usually takes longer to reduce heart attack risk by lowering cholesterol. Many foods do both, however, such as onions and garlic, so you get double benefits.

"Everybody knows it is not cholesterol that kills you. It's the blood clot that forms on top of the cholesterol-hardened plaque in the arteries that can be deadly."

—Dr. David Kritchevsky,
Wistar Institute, Philadelphia

Cardiologists once thought the narrowing of arteries from plaque buildup triggered heart attacks by leading to heart rhythm disturbances. But it's now widely accepted that a blood clot is the immediate cause of 80 to 90 percent of heart attacks as well as strokes. Several factors, strongly affected by diet, are critical to whether or not you form clots. One is how prone your platelets—the smallest of blood cells—are to aggregate or clump together, enabling them to form clots and better cling to vessel walls. Another factor: blood fibrinogen, a protein that is a raw material for clot formation. High circulating levels of fibrinogen are prime predictors of heart disease and stroke.

Also crucial is your *fibrinolytic* system, which breaks up and dissolves unwanted and dangerous clots. The vigor of this clot-dissolving activity along with fibrinogen levels is the "number one determinant of heart disease," says Harvard cardiologist Dr. Victor Gurewich.

How Food Can Control Blood Clotting

Doctors routinely warn against taking aspirin before surgery. The fear is that aspirin can "thin the blood," slowing blood clotting. Therefore, you may bleed longer, causing complications and jeopardizing your recovery, when you need rapid blood clotting to plug the wound made by the scalpel.

But did you ever have a surgeon tell you not to eat Chinese food before an operation? Or to avoid heavy doses of ginger, garlic, black mushrooms, and fatty fish like salmon and sardines? The truth is that all of these foods are also anticoagulants that may dramatically retard blood-clotting tendencies and often by exactly the same biological mechanism as aspirin—by blocking a substance called thromboxane that clamps down on platelet clumping or aggregation, a crucial step in clot formation.

In contrast, fatty foods like cheese and steak cause the blood to become sluggish by making platelets stickier and more apt to clot.

Additionally, certain foods raise or lower blood

clot-essential fibrinogen and rev up or slow down the clot-dissolving activity. Still other foods influence blood viscosity and fluidity, setting the stage for or staving off inappropriate clots that can cause blood vessel blockages in the heart, brain, legs, and lungs. Undeniably, foods in very small quantities regularly eaten can have powerful pharmacological effects on the tendency of blood to clot, and thus, can help save you from cardiovascular tragedies.

One of your greatest weapons—if not your primary one—against heart attack and stroke is to eat foods that benefit blood-clotting factors. Here's what to eat and not to eat.

Garlic and Onions: Ancient Clot Fighters

It's an ancient truth: garlic and onions are strong medicines against unwanted blood clots. An early Egyptian papyrus called onions a tonic for the blood. Early American doctors prescribed onions as "blood purifiers." French farmers feed horses garlic and onions to dissolve blood clots in their legs. The Russians claim vodka spiked with garlic improves circulation. It's no longer unsubstantiated folklore. Garlic and onions are full of potent clot-fighting compounds and powers.

Eric Block, Ph.D., head of the chemistry department at the State University of New York at Albany, isolated a garlic compound named ajoene (after *ajo*, the Spanish word for garlic) that has antithrombotic activity, equal to or exceeding that of aspirin, a well-recognized blood clot inhibitor. Indeed, aspirin performs only one way as an anticoagulant by stifling production of thromboxane. Ajoene does that, and additionally blocks platelet clumping seven other ways—by all pathways known, according to garlic researcher Mahendra K. Jain, Ph.D., professor of chemistry and biochemistry at the University of Delaware. "Garlic's mechanism is unique," he says.

"Clinical studies seem to be pretty much in agreement that there's something in garlic that helps prevent blood clotting."

—Eric Block, Ph.D.,
State University of New York at Albany

George Washington University medical researchers have detected three additional anticlotting compounds in garlic and onions, including a major one, adenosine.

Garlic's antithrombotic activity in humans is well documented by numerous studies. Three raw garlic cloves a day recently improved both clotting time and clot-dissolving fibrinolytic activity by about 20 percent in a double-blind study of fifty medical students in India.

Recent German research shows that garlic compounds definitely speed up blood clot dissolving activity and improve blood fluidity. Such simultaneous action, researchers at Saarland University in Homburg/Saar say, improves circulation and in fact helps "purify" the blood of unwanted elements.

How much garlic? Only one or two cloves of garlic have a pronounced beneficial effect on clotting activity, says David Roser, a British garlic researcher.

Note: You can eat garlic raw or cooked to discourage blood clots. The bulb's antithrombotic effects are not destroyed by heat; in fact, they can be released by cooking.

Onions: A Potent Fat Blocker

To help keep blood free of clots, eat onions, both raw and cooked. Harvard's Dr. Victor Gurewich advises all his patients with coronary heart disease to eat onions daily, partly because their compounds hinder platelet clumping and speed up clot-dissolving activity. In fact, onions have a truly astonishing ability to counteract the detrimental clot-promoting effects of eating fatty foods. N. N. Gupta, professor of medicine at K. G. Medical College in Lucknow, India, first fed men a very high fat meal, with butter and cream, and commissioned that their clot-dissolving activity plunged.

Then he gave them the same fatty meal, this time adding two ounces of onions, raw, boiled, or fried. Blood drawn two and four hours after the fatty meal showed that the onions had totally blocked the fat's detrimental blood-clotting proclivities. Indeed, less than half a cup of onions completely reversed the fat's damaging effects on clot-dissolving activity.

What is it about onions that helps prevent clots? It could be quercetin, a formidable antioxidant with wide-ranging activity, concentrated in onions. It helps block formation of blood clots and processes that lead to artery clogging. In a Finnish study, those eating the most bioflavonoids, mainly quercetin, were least likely to suffer fatal heart attacks. For the most quercetin, eat red and yellow onions; white onions have very little. Coming soon: super-potent onions. At the University of Wisconsin and the University of Texas M.D. Anderson Cancer Center, researchers are developing onions extra-high in quercetin and other disease-fighting phytochemicals. Red wine, broccoli, and tea are also rich in quercetin.

- **BOTTOM LINE:** When you eat fatty foods, add some onions. That slice of onion on a hamburger or those onions in your omelet or on your pizza may help counteract the clot-promoting powers of the fatty foods.

Dr. Jain's Blood-Thinning Garlic Tips

One of garlic's most powerful and well-tested anti-coagulant compounds is called ajoene. Here are some ways to release the most ajoene from garlic, according to garlic researcher Mahendra K. Jain, Ph.D., professor of biochemistry at the University of Delaware.

- Crush garlic instead of chopping it. Crushing releases enzymes and the allicin that converts to ajoene.
- Sauté garlic lightly; cooking releases ajoene.
- Cook garlic with tomatoes or add to other acidic foods. Even a little acid releases ajoene.
- Add just enough vodka to cover crushed garlic, and let steep for several days uncovered. This releases ajoene. Yes, the old Russian folk recipe for this blood-thinning potion really works, Dr. Jain's tests revealed. He also found that mixing crushed garlic with feta cheese and olive oil, which is a reputed Greek remedy for heart disease, produced lots of ajoene.

How About a Little Fish Pâté?

For a clot blocker and clot buster, you can't beat fish, high in the marvelous omega-3 fatty acids. Most scientists attribute fish's heart-protecting powers primarily to the oil's remarkable effects on blood coagulation. Studies consistently show that fish oil regulates how the blood flows and clots. Since 80 percent of strokes stem from blood clots, eating oily fish may act as a mild anticoagulant to thwart formation of dangerous clots. For example, men who eat a mere three-quarters of an ounce or more of fish a day have half the risk of stroke as non-fish eaters, according to a recent Dutch study. The probable reason, say researchers: fewer blood clots.

When you eat fatty fish such as salmon, mackerel, herring, sardines, tuna, or indeed any fish containing some fat, it launches multiple attacks against clots: the oil tends to thin the blood by suppressing platelet clumping, depressing fibrinogen, and revving up clot-dissolving activity. Paul Nestel, chief of Human Nutrition at the Commonwealth Scientific and Industrial Research Organization in Australia, and his colleagues have found that eating about five ounces of salmon or sardines a day lowered hazardous fibrinogen an average 16 percent and prolonged bleeding time by 11 percent in a group of thirty-one men. Interestingly, in the same study, fish oil capsules did *not* affect blood-clotting factors. One explanation, says Dr. Nestel, is that fish have other compounds besides fat that benefit anticlotting factors.

Similarly, Harvard researchers suggested that eating six and a half ounces of canned tuna could "thin the blood" as much as taking an aspirin. The anticlotting effects came about four hours after eating the tuna. Also, subjects absorbed more of the oils from tuna than from fish oil capsules.

Fish Oil's Remarkable "Blood-Thinning" Secret

Eating fatty fish literally changes the shape of blood platelets so they can't lock together to form unwanted blood clots. That's what researchers at the U.S. Department of Agriculture discovered. When you eat fish oil, your platelets release much less of the substance called thromboxane that instructs platelets to stick together, according to USDA's Norberta Schoene, Ph.D.

More fascinating, thromboxane creates sticky platelets by stimulating them to swell up into little round balloons and then to grow spikes so that they can interlock with other platelets. In this state they are "activated," or "sticky," ready and able to clump together to form blood clots.

Thus, fatty fish, by suppressing thromboxane, preserves the healthy normal disk shape of platelets so they can't cling together and form clots to plug up your arteries.

- **BOTTOM LINE:** You get a favorable antithrombotic effect from eating about three and a half ounces of fatty fish—such as mackerel, herring, salmon, and sardines—or about six ounces of canned tuna.

Red Wine's Wondrous Anticoagulant

A little red wine can often thin your blood, retarding clots. The reason is not just the alcohol but other complex constituents in the red wine. In a classic study, the French scientists Martine Seigneur and Jacques Bonnet, M.D., at the Hospital Cardiologique in Pessac, tested the effects of three alcoholic beverages on blood clotting in fifteen healthy men. Every day for two weeks they drank a half liter of either a red Bordeaux wine, a white Bordeaux wine, or a synthetic wine made with water, alcohol, and flavorings. The results: The synthetic wine increased platelet clumping and decreased bad LDL cholesterol. White wine slightly boosted detrimental LDLs and markedly increased benevolent HDLs, but did not change platelets. Red wine was the clear winner! It both depressed platelet clumping and boosted HDL cholesterol. Thus, the researchers pronounced red wine's anticoagulant powers unique in protecting the heart.

Their findings are backed by French studies in animals showing that detrimental blood-clotting activity (platelet stickiness or aggregation) was initially depressed by red wine, white wine, and straight alcohol. Fourteen hours later, however, investigators detected a "rebound effect" from white wine and alcohol. Blood-clotting tendency from red wine was still down about 60 percent, but blood stickiness had shot up 46 percent in white wine drinkers and 124 percent in those who drank plain alcohol.

One type of white wine, however, champagne, may be an exception; it appears to have antioxidant, anti-clogging benefit, says Dr. Serge Renaud, famed French government researcher. He explains that the antioxidant-containing grape skins are often left in the mix longer when making champagne than when making other white wines.

On the other side of the Atlantic, Dr. John Folts at the University of Wisconsin-Madison Medical School, found that drinking two and a half glasses of red wine reduced blood platelet stickiness and thus the tendency to form hazardous clots by 40 percent within forty-five minutes. Purple grape juice also works, he says, but it takes three times as much grape juice as red wine for the same anticoagulant benefit.

What accounts for the anti-blood-clotting effects of wine and grape juice? The French said they were not sure they wanted to know, nor did they want the compound isolated, insisting that "the medicine is already in a highly palatable form." Cornell University scientists have suggested that wine's main anticlotting agent is resveratrol, a chemical in grape skins. Other researchers have identified nitric oxide and several other antioxidants called polyphenols or flavonoids in red wine and grapes that they credit for the clot-fighting activity.

Why Grapes Make Anticlotting Medicine

Rejoice in a grape's misfortune. Every time a grape is attacked by fungal infection, it defends itself by spinning out a natural pesticide somewhat the way humans make antibodies to combat infections. This plant pesticide is also a glorious anti-blood-clotting medication. The compound, say Japanese researchers, is the main active ingredient in an ancient Chinese and Japanese folk medicine used to treat blood disorders. Indeed, the Japanese have concentrated this grape compound, resveratrol, into a drug, and in tests have found it hinders blood platelet clumping that leads to blood clots and reduces fatty deposits in animal livers.

If you drink red grape juice or red wine you may get some resveratrol, says Leroy Creasy, Ph.D., a professor at Cornell University's College of Agriculture. Dr. Creasy detected high concentrations of the anticlotting substance in red wine, but not in white wine. His explanation: In making red wine, crushed grapes are left to sit with the skins to ferment. But in making white wine, the grapes are pressed and the resveratrol-rich skins discarded. Dr. Creasy's analysis of thirty types of wine found the most resveratrol in a red French Bordeaux and the least in a white Bordeaux.

Dr. Creasy also found the anticoagulant in purple (but not white) grape juice. He also figures it takes about three times as much grape juice as red Bordeaux wine to get equal amounts of the compound. Table grapes found in supermarkets probably contain little of the substance because they are carefully cultivated to prevent fungal infections and blemishes. A pound of homegrown grapes, however, can have as much resveratrol as two cups of red wine, says Dr. Creasy.

- **BOTTOM LINE:** Regular intake of red wine, in moderation with meals, seems to promote antithrombotic activity, discouraging heart disease. That means one glass of wine per day for women and two for men. Heavier drinking and binge drinking can encourage blood clotting and cardiovascular damage, and may increase a woman's risk of breast cancer. It's important to drink the red wine with meals so it can directly cancel out clot-promoting factors in the rest of the meal.

Drink Tea for Healthy Arteries

Curious as it may seem, drinking tea gives your arteries an antithrombotic infusion. In 1967 the British scientific journal *Nature* carried some extraordinary photos of the aortas of rabbits given a high-fat, high-cholesterol diet plus either water or tea to drink. The aortas of the tea-drinking rabbits were much less scarred and ravaged by the high-fat diet. Tea, concluded the researchers from Lawrence-Livermore Labs in California, had prevented much of the arterial damage. They were inspired to do the experiments after noticing that the arteries of Chinese-Americans who regularly drank tea exhibited only two-thirds as much coronary artery damage and only one-third as much cerebral artery damage at autopsy as Caucasian coffee drinkers. Their suggestion that mysterious compounds in tea could keep blood vessels from clogging was ahead of its time.

Science has caught up. Research presented at the first international scientific conference on the physiological and pharmacological effects of tea, held in New York City in 1991, reveals that tea protects arteries by influencing blood-clotting factors. Tea chemicals can reduce blood coagulability, preventing platelet activation and clumping, increase clot-dissolving activity, and decrease deposits of cholesterol in artery walls—all of which help fend off artery damage. In animal research, giving the equivalent of three cups of tea for a human reduced platelet clumping and prevented blood clotting.

A pioneer in tea and atherosclerosis, Lou Fu-qing, M.D., professor and chairman of the Department of Internal Medicine at Zhejiang Medical University in China, has studied the effect of tea chemicals on heart attack victims. Dr. Lou told the conference that pigment from common black tea or Asian style green tea thwarted patients' platelet clumping (also thromboxane production) and improved their clot-dissolving functioning. Surprisingly, he said both ordinary black tea that Americans commonly drink and Asian green tea worked equally well. Scientists at Japan's Ito-en Central Research Institute also noted that a particular type of tannin in green tea, called catechin, blocked the clumping of platelets just as strongly as aspirin did. Tea also appears to help block LDL cholesterol's stimulation of the proliferation of smooth muscle cells on the walls of arteries; such cell growth fosters the buildup of arterial plaque.

Vegetables Are Clot Busters

To discourage unwanted blood clots, eat fruits and vegetables high in vitamin C and fiber. The most prodigious eaters of fruits and vegetables have the most energetic clot-dissolving systems, according to a Swedish study of 260 middle-aged adults. Those who ate the least fruits and vegetables had the most sluggish clot-dissolving activity. Other studies show that vitamin C and fiber, concentrated in fruits and vegetables, also rev up clot-dissolving mechanisms and help thwart platelet clumping that leads to clots.

Further, the lowest levels of clot-promoting fibrinogen belong to vegetarians, especially vegans who eat no animal products at all, including eggs and milk. The probable reason is that compounds in fruits and vegetables lower fibrinogen, while animal fat and cholesterol push it up. Vegetarians also have lower blood viscosity than meat eaters; lower viscosity is linked to lower blood pressure. So it's one more way fruits and vegetables ward off heart disease.

The Hot Chili Pepper Effect

Hot chili peppers are clot busters. Evidence for this comes from Thailand, where citizens eat capsicum chili peppers as a seasoning and as an appetizer, infusing their blood with chili pepper compounds several times a day. Thai researchers reasoned that this may be a primary reason thromboembolisms—life threatening blood clots—are rare among Thais.

To prove the theory, hematologist Sukon Visudhiphan, M.D., and colleagues at the Siriraj Hospital in Bangkok did a test. They fortified homemade rice noodles with hot pepper, using two teaspoons of fresh ground capsicum jalapeño pepper in every 200 grams of noodles (about one and one-third cups). Then they fed the peppery noodles to sixteen healthy medical students. The other, control subjects ate plain noodles. Almost immediately, the clot-dissolving activity of the blood of the eaters of pepper-laced noodles rose, but returned to normal in about thirty minutes. Nothing happened to the blood of the plain noodle eaters.

The chili pepper effect was short-lived. However, Dr. Visudhiphan believes the frequent stimulation from hot chilis continually clears the blood of clots, leaving Thais generally less vulnerable to arterial blockage.

Spicy Clot Busters

Eat common spices to keep your blood free of dangerous clots. Krishna Srivastava, of Odense University in Denmark, screened eleven spices and found that seven discouraged blood platelet clumping. Most potent are cloves, ginger, cumin, and tumeric. "Cloves are stronger than aspirin in this respect," says Dr. Srivastava. The primary active agent in cloves is probably eugenol, which also helps protect the structure of platelets even after they have been "aggregated." Dr. Srivastava says the spices work through the prostaglandin system, somewhat the way aspirin, garlic, and onions do.

For example, all the spices clamped down on production of thromboxane, which is a potent promoter of platelet clumping. Ginger compounds are a stronger inhibitor of prostaglandin synthesis than the drug indomethacin, known for its potency, says Dr. Srivastava.

Ginger is indeed a proven anticoagulant in humans, as Charles R. Dorso, M.D., of the Cornell University Medical College, discovered after eating a large quantity of Crabtree & Evelyn Ginger with Grapefruit Marmalade, which was 15 percent ginger. When his blood did not coagulate as usual, he did a test by mixing some ground ginger with his own blood platelets, and found them less sticky. Dr. Dorso said the active agent is gingerol, a constituent of ginger, that chemically resembles aspirin.

Cautions: If your stomach hurts after eating spicy foods, avoid them. If you take anticoagulants, consult a doctor before adding large amounts of potentially blood-thinning ginger.

Black Mushrooms:
A Sure Blood Thinner

To ward off clots, infuse your blood with the medicine of the Asian black fungus mushroom known as *mo-er*, or "tree ear." It has a formidable reputation in Chinese traditional medicine for its beneficial effects on blood. Some call it a "longevity tonic." With good reason, according to Dale Hammerschmidt, M.D., a hematologist at the University of Minnesota Medical School. He once ate a large quantity of *mapo doufu*, a spicy Asian bean curd dish containing the mushrooms, and afterward noticed dramatic changes in how his blood platelets behaved. They were much less apt to clump. He traced the anticoagulant effect to the black mushrooms.

It turns out that the black mushrooms (but not ordinary button mushrooms) contain several blood-thinning compounds, including adenosine, also present in garlic and onions. Dr. Hammerschmidt surmises that the combination of so many anticlotting foods in the

Chinese diet—such as garlic, onions, black mushrooms, and ginger—may help account for their low rates of coronary artery disease.

Olive Oil Fights Clots

In addition to everything else it does, olive oil even retards the stickiness of blood platelets, which may help account for olive oil's artery-protecting powers. For example, British researchers at the Royal Free Hospital and School of Medicine in London had volunteers take three-fourths of a tablespoon of olive oil twice a day for eight weeks in addition to their regular diet. Their platelet-clumping scores took a dive. The scientists found that platelet membranes contained more oleic acid (the dominant fatty acid in olive oil), and less arachidonic fatty acid that encourages stickiness.

The olive-oil-fed blood platelets also released less thromboxane A2, a substance that commands platelets to cling together. All told, olive oil benefits platelet function, the researchers concluded, saying it is yet one more explanation of why populations that depend heavily on olive oil—in the Mediterranean area—have less heart disease.

High Fat—Blood Clot Villain

Go easy on fat if you want to keep your blood clear of clots. Unquestionably, a high-fat diet does bad things to your blood beyond boosting your blood cholesterol. Too much fat can also buck up the blood's tendency to coagulate and form dangerous clots. A recent study by researchers at South Jutland University Center in Denmark, for example, found that high amounts of both saturated animal type fat and certain omega-6 polyunsaturated vegetable fats, such as corn oil, promoted clot-forming fibrinogen. In their study, a group of healthy adults who ordinarily ate high-fat diets switched to various lower-fat diets (32 percent of calories) for two weeks at a time. All the low-fat diets suppressed blood-clotting tendencies by 10 to 15 percent. Much research also shows that fat, particularly animal fat, slows down clot-dissolving activity.

One recent study found that the fat from a fatty meal lingers in the bloodstream, fomenting trouble, for up to four hours.

Try a Clot-Busting Breakfast

It's long been a mystery why most heart attacks happen within a few hours after the victim wakes up in the morning. One reason may be that people skip breakfast, suggests research by cardiologist Renata Cifkova of the Memorial University of Newfoundland in St. Johns. She found that skipping breakfast nearly triples your clot-forming potential, leaving you more vulnerable to heart attacks and strokes. Dr. Cifkova explains that blood platelet stickiness is lowest overnight, then climbs rapidly when you wake up. But for mysterious reasons, eating seems to "unstick" the platelets.

As proof, she measured a marker of platelet activity called beta-thromboglobulin (beta-TG) in the blood of twenty-nine normal men and women on days they ate or skipped breakfast. Beta-TG indicates blood platelet potential for clotting. She found that the beta-TG averaged two and a half times higher on the day the group skipped breakfast. However, the beta-TG dropped markedly on the days when they ate breakfast. Thus, it appears that one way to keep your blood platelets from remaining dangerously sticky, and putting you in morning heart attack territory, is to break your fast when you get up—eat breakfast.

Diet Advice to Combat Blood Clots

Eating to control your blood-clotting factors is probably the most important dietary measure you can take to ward off coronary heart disease and strokes—even more important than controlling cholesterol. Here are your best bets:

- Eat fatty fish, garlic, onions, ginger, and red wine (in moderation). All may help to thin the blood and keep blood from forming inappropriate clots.
- Restrict fat, notably saturated animal fat and omega-6 type polyunsaturated fats, to discourage blood clots.
- Make it a point to eat clot-discouraging foods at the same time you eat foods that can encourage clotting. Some winning combinations are eggs and onions or lox, red wine and cheese, hot peppers and chili con carne.

Caution: Don't go overboard. If you are on blood-thinning medications, have bleeding problems or have a family history of "bleeding" or hemorrhagic stroke, you should be moderate about foods that thin the blood. If concerned, have your doctor check your blood to be sure it is clotting normally.

Chapter 4

Nature's Strong Medicine Against Strokes

Foods That Help Prevent Strokes or Lessen Damage: Fruits • Vegetables • Seafood, Especially Fatty Fish • Tea • A Little Alcohol
Foods That May Promote Strokes: Salt • Excessive Alcohol • Saturated Animal Fats

As you grow older, your odds of having a stroke rise steadily. Yet, there is dramatic evidence that what you eat can slash your chances of stroke as well as the damage it may cause, and even help determine whether or not it is fatal. About 80 percent of strokes among Americans are due to clots in blood vessels of the brain and head. The rest come from hemorrhages or "bleeding strokes" when vessels rupture, spilling blood into the brain. Thus, foods that help ward off clots keep blood vessels flexible and unclogged, and keep blood pressure normal are good bets for preventing strokes. Even one extra daily portion of the right stuff may cut an astounding 40 to 60 percent or even more off your chances of having or dying of a stroke. Any drug that promised to prevent that many strokes a year would be an overnight sensation, despite its cost and potential side effects. Yet, such an effective and certainly safer and cheaper drug is in everyone's possession right now.

Nature's Brain Protectors

The "right stuff" to keep strokes away is fruits and vegetables, according to overwhelming evidence. More than a decade ago, researchers discovered that eating fruits and vegetables prevented strokes and diminished the damage if they occurred. British researchers at Cambridge University discovered that older people who ate the most fresh green vegetables and fresh fruits were less apt to die of strokes. A Norwegian study found that men who ate the most vegetables had a 45 percent lower risk of stroke. It also found that women who ate lots of fruit were one-third less likely to have a stroke.

Since then the evidence has piled up. The famous Framingham Heart study noted that men who ate the most fruit and vegetables were least apt to have a stroke or warning sign of stroke—a TIA (transient ischemic attack). Adding only three servings of fruits and vegetables per day reduced stroke risk 22 percent. Dutch researchers found that those who ate the most flavonoids—antioxidants in fruits, vegetables, and tea—slashed their risk of stroke by 73 percent.

Stroke Survival Medicine: An Extra Carrot a Day

Imagine! Eating carrots five times a week or more could slash your risk of stroke by an astounding two-thirds, or 68 percent, compared with eating carrots but once a month or less! That's the dramatic finding of a recent large-scale Harvard study that tracked nearly 90,000 women nurses for eight years. Spinach was also a particularly potent stroke deterrent. Part of the protection comes from beta carotene in carrots and spinach. A previous Harvard study found that eating the extra beta carotene in about one and a half carrots, three-fourths of a cup of mashed sweet potatoes, or three cups of cooked spinach every day shaved 40 percent off stroke rates. The drop was evident in those who ate 15 to 20 milligrams of beta carotene daily versus those who ate only 6 milligrams.

What gives carrots, spinach, and other such carotene-rich vegetables antistroke activity is probably their antioxidant activity, speculated lead researcher JoAnn E. Manson, M.D., of Brigham and Women's Hospital and Harvard Medical School. The carotene inhibits cholesterol from becoming toxic and able to form plaque and clots in arteries, she theorized.

More remarkable is new research showing how important it is to have lots of beta carotene and other vitamin A in your bloodstream should you ever suffer a stroke. The vitamin may prevent your death or disability from the stroke, according to Belgian researchers at the University of Brussels, who analyzed the blood of eighty patients within twenty-four hours after they had suffered strokes. They discovered that stroke patients with above-average amounts of vitamin A, including beta carotene, were more apt to survive, to have less neurologic damage, and to recover completely! Here's why: When your brain is deprived of oxygen, as in a stroke, cells begin to malfunction, leading to a series of events culminating in oxidative damage to nerve cells. But if you have lots of vitamin A in your blood, researchers speculate, it can interfere at many different stages of this cascade of events, lessening brain damage and chances of death.

Foods rich in beta carotene—also known as vegetable vitamin A because it converts in the body to vitamin A—in addition to carrots are dark green leafy vegetables such as spinach, collards, and kale, as well as dark orange vegetables such as sweet potatoes and pumpkin. Such foods are also high in potassium, another potent antidote against strokes.

The Remarkable California Experiment

Eat just one extra serving of a potassium-rich food every day; that too may reduce your risk of stroke by 40 percent. That's what researchers discovered by analyzing the diets of a group of 859 men and women over age 50 living in southern California. The investigators documented that small differences in potassium in the diet predicted who would die of a stroke twelve years later.

Remarkably, nobody with the highest intake of potassium (more than 3,500 milligrams a day) died of a stroke. However, those who regularly ate the least potassium (less than 1,950 milligrams per day) had much higher fatal stroke rates than all the others. Among those who skimped the most on potassium, the odds of stroke deaths shot up 2.6 times in men and 4.8 times in women. Further, the more potassium-rich foods the subjects ate, generally the fewer strokes they had. Indeed, the researchers concluded that with every extra daily 400 milligrams of potassium in food, the odds of a fatal stroke dropped 40 percent!

That critical margin of 400 milligrams of potassium is so modest, you find it in a single piece of most fruits and vegetables, a glass of milk, or a small chunk of fish. If you thought it would help protect your brain from that devastating and often irreversible human catastrophe known as stroke or cerebrovascular accident, wouldn't it be worth it to eat every day an extra quarter of a cantaloupe, half an avocado, one small baked potato, ten dried apricots, a half cup of baked beans, or a small tin of sardines?

High-potassium foods help lower blood pressure, but potassium exhibits additional powers to prevent stroke directly regardless of blood pressure, says University of Minnesota hypertension expert Dr. Louis Tobian Jr. In tests, he fed rats that had high blood pressure either a high-potassium diet or a "normal" potassium diet. Forty percent on the "normal" potassium regimen suffered small strokes, evidenced by bleeding in the brain. No brain hemorrhages occurred in rats on high potassium. Dr. Tobian's theory is that extra potassium kept artery walls elastic and functioning normally, thus immunizing blood vessels against damage from high blood pressure. The same thing may happen in humans.

Fatty Fish—The Blood Fixers

Another spectacular thing you can do for blood circulation in your brain is to eat fatty fish. The omega-3 type fatty acids in fish perform several miracles on blood that make strokes less likely to occur. For one, these fats act as a mild anticoagulant to thwart formation of dangerous clots. And even if a stroke happens, the damage is apt to be less if you have high levels of such fatty acids in your blood. Even eating a little fish may save you from stroke. Recent Dutch research found that men between the ages of 60 and 69 who ate fish at least once a week were only half as apt to have a stroke during the next fifteen years as those who ate no fish. The probable reason, say researchers: fewer blood clots.

Further, a series of studies in Japan show that heavy fish eaters are less apt to die if they have a stroke. Researchers found 25 to 40 percent fewer *fatal* strokes in farmers who ate only three ounces of fish a day.

It's also well established that the marvelous omega-3 fat in fish can modify the blood, making it less prone to clotting, obviously discouraging blockage in cere-

What People Eat Who Don't Die of Strokes

Each of these foods provides the extra 400 milligrams of daily potassium shown to slash the odds of fatal stroke by 40 percent:

- 1/2 cup cooked fresh spinach (423 milligrams)
- 1/2 cup cooked fresh beet greens (654 milligrams)
- 1 teaspoon blackstrap molasses (400 milligrams)
- 1 cup tomato juice (536 milligrams)
- 1 cup fresh orange juice (472 milligrams)
- 1/4 cantaloupe (412 milligrams)
- 1/2 cup acorn squash (446 milligrams)
- 10 dried apricot halves (482 milligrams)
- 2 carrots (466 milligrams)
- 1/2 cup cooked sweet potato (455 milligrams)
- 1/2 cup cooked green lima beans (484 milligrams)
- 1 cup skim milk (418 milligrams)
- 1/2 Florida avocado (742 milligrams)
- 1 banana (451 milligrams)
- 2 ounces almonds (440 milligrams)
- 1 ounce roasted soybeans (417 milligrams)
- 17-ounce baked potato without skin (512 milligrams)

- 17-ounce baked potato with skin
  (844 milligrams)
- 1/2 cup baked beans (613 milligrams)
- 3 ounces (about eight) canned sardines
  (500 milligrams)
- 3 ounces swordfish steak (465 milligrams)

bral blood vessels. Some remarkable pioneering studies by William Lands, Ph.D., then at the University of
Illinois in Chicago, showed that damage from strokes
in animals was considerably less if they had previously eaten fish oils. If you are at the age where you fear
your capillaries are narrowed by plaque buildup, here
is an image to treasure: When you eat fish oil, it set-
tles in the structural membranes of your cells. Such
cells, when full of fish oil, are less stiff, more fluid and
pliable. This means such deformable blood cells are
better able to squeeze through constricted blood vessels, supplying brain cells and heart cells with oxygen.
Such maneuverability could be lifesaving, especially
as your arteries age and narrow.

Incidentally, eating saturated animal fat tends to
make cell membranes more rigid. It's one more reason
for those worried about stroke and cardiovascular disease in general to shun such fat.

Saved by Tea

Deflect strokes by drinking tea, both black and green tea. In a long-running Dutch study, men who drank the most black tea had a much lower incidence of stroke than those drinking the least amount of tea. And a four-year study of nearly 6,000 women over age 40, by Japanese physicians at Tohoku University School of Medicine, found that women who drank at least five cups of green tea every day were only half as likely to suffer a stroke as those who drank less. It was also true for women with high salt intake, who typically have increased risk of high blood pressure and stroke. The study is the first of its kind to link green tea directly with stroke prevention, although earlier animal studies in Japan, China, and the United States found that green tea decreases blood pressure.

One explanation for the antistroke activity may be the high concentration of antioxidants in tea, which might protect blood vessels from damage. One study found green tea chemicals even stronger in antioxidant effect than vitamins E and C, well known for their potent antioxidant powers. Tea may also ward off stroke by preventing blood clots; compounds called flavonoids, present in tea, also have a modest anticlotting effect.

New Salt Danger

Beware salt. Even if it does not raise your blood pressure, it may nevertheless be detrimental to brain tissue, helping induce ministrokes, says Dr. Tobian. He came to this conclusion after tests in which he fed rats either a high-salt or a low-salt diet. The high-salt diet induced deadly strokes in the animals even though it did not raise their blood pressure. Within fifteen weeks, an astonishing 100 percent of the high-salt-fed animals were dead, compared with only 12 percent of the low-salt animals. The brains of the dead rats on high-salt diets revealed injured arteries and dead tissue, caused by a series of fatal ministrokes.

Dr. Tobian advises cutting back on salt to avoid stroke even if salt does not boost your blood pressure. This is especially critical for people over age 65 and all African-Americans, two groups especially vulnerable to salt's damage, he says.

Added Iron Danger

Excessive iron may accelerate artery destruction. Neurologists at University Clinic in Innsbruck, Austria, compared the amount of blockage of carotid (neck) arteries in 847 men and women. They found that high stores of iron (ferritin) in tissues was "one of the strongest indicator of carotid artery disease" in both men and women ages 40 to 70. The Austrian researchers also found more extensive carotid artery clogging in men than in women until after age 70— possibly, they said, because men store more iron than menstruating women.

To avoid excessive iron, add up the iron in your supplements and fortified cereal and make sure you're not exceeding the recommended levels for your age and sex group. Postmenopausal women and men of any age don't need more than 10 milligrams daily. Premenopausal women need a daily 15 mg. The exception: anyone diagnosed with iron-deficiency anemia. In that case, consult with your doctor about how much supplementary iron to take, and stop taking high levels once the anemia is reversed. Also, limit your intake of red meat, which is high in iron.

Alcohol:
Good News, Bad News

Light to moderate drinking could help save you from a stroke, but heavy drinking may bring on a stroke, according to new evidence from Columbia University in New York City. This study compared 677 multiethnic people age 40 and over who had already suffered one ischemic (blood clot–induced) stroke with a similar group who hadn't had strokes. They found that those who drank moderately, defined as up to two drinks a day, were at 45 percent lower risk of having a stroke than nondrinkers. However, those who drank heavily—seven or more drinks a day—increased their stroke risk threefold.

Studies worldwide show the same thing. For instance, Italian and Austrian neurologists who studied the drinking habits of 826 men and women showed that an alcoholic drink a day may help prevent fatty deposits that lead to heart attack and stroke. But more than four daily drinks increase the risk of stroke even more than heavy smoking does. The heaviest drinkers were most apt to have fatty buildup in vessels leading to the brain, setting the stage for stroke. British researchers documented that those consuming a drink or two a day were only 60 to 70 percent as vulnerable as nondrinkers to either a hemorrhagic (bleeding) stroke or clot-induced stroke. On the other hand, heavy drinkers—three to four drinks a day—were three times more prone to strokes than nondrinkers.

Worse, a University of Helsinki study found heavy drinkers six times more susceptible to strokes! Alcohol, the Finnish neurologists remind us, is a brain poison, and in heavy doses promotes brain embolisms, clots, and ischemia due to blood changes and contraction of blood vessels—all preludes to strokes. The Finns also found that moderate drinkers were much less likely to suffer strokes than nondrinkers!

Wine may be the best way to go, according to a long-term study by Danish researchers at the Institute of Preventive Medicine in Copenhagen. They found that drinking a beer or more a day boosted the risk of having a stroke by 9 percent. But moderately drinking wine, a little less than a glass a day, lowered stroke risk by 34 percent. Researchers credited antioxidants concentrated in red wine. Two-thirds of the wine consumed in Denmark is red.

Besides the antioxidants in red wine, alcohol itself has anti-inflammatory activity, research shows. This is important because researchers now believe inflammation of blood vessels contributes to plaque buildup and consequently to heart disease, strokes, and possibly Alzheimer's disease. Further, National Institutes of Health researchers recently reported that moderate drinkers have less rheumatoid arthritis, an inflammatory disease.

- **BOTTOM LINE:** A drink or two a day, if you already drink, may be beneficial, but you should not take up drinking to try to avert a stroke. Heavy drinkers should take heed and cut back, for few events are more tragic than a stroke.

An Antistroke Diet Prescription

It seems urgent and clear: If you are worried about a stroke, do the following six things:

1. Eat lots of fruits and vegetables, five or more servings a day. Be sure to include carrots, and folic acid–rich orange juice and dark leafy greens.
2. Eat fish, especially fatty fish, at least three times a week.
3. Watch your sodium intake.
4. Don't drink alcohol excessively—no more than a drink or two a day.

5. Consider drinking tea—either green tea or ordinary black tea brewed from tea bags or loose tea. Bottled teas and instant tea mixes do not contain heart-protective antioxidants, according to research at the U.S. Department of Agriculture.
6. Eat fat in moderation; don't go on an extremely low fat diet.

Remember, such actions could also curb neurological damage and lower your odds of dying if you do have a stroke.

Chapter 5

Diet Remedies for High Blood Pressure

Foods That May Lower Blood Pressure: Celery • Garlic • Fatty Fish • Fruits • Vegetables • Olive Oil • High-Calcium Foods • High-Potassium Foods • High-Fiber Foods
Foods That May Raise Blood Pressure: High-Sodium Foods • Alcohol

Your blood pressure is a major marker of heart health, and keeping it normal—not in excess of 140/90 by American standards—unquestionably helps ward off heart attacks and strokes. You can take pharmacological drugs, of course; you can also get drugs in foods that possess surprising power to lower blood pressure. Much research shows that foods are laden with blood pressure boosters and reducers. Eating your way out of high blood pressure is increasingly the number one choice of virtually all experts, in lieu of or in addition to pharmacological drugs. Try diet first. The list of foods that may help lower blood pressure is growing longer and capturing the attention and imaginations of ever more mainstream physicians.

Try Celery, an Ancient Medicine

Celery has been used as a folk remedy to lower blood pressure in Asian cultures since 200 B.C., says William J. Elliott, a pharmacologist at the University of Chicago's Pritzker School of Medicine, who recently isolated a blood pressure–reducing drug in celery. Dr. Elliott became intrigued when Vietnamese graduate student Quang T. Le mentioned that his father's high blood pressure had been successfully treated by a traditional Asian doctor who prescribed celery. After Minh Le, 62 years old, ate two stalks of celery every day for a week, his blood pressure dropped from a high 158/96 to a normal 118/82.

Dr. Elliott made an "educated guess" about what chemical in celery might lower blood pressure. He extracted the compound and gave it to rats with normal blood pressure. It worked. Their systolic (upper number) blood pressure sank an average 12 to 14 percent when the animals were given celery extract for a couple of weeks. The doses were comparable to eating four stalks a day. Their blood cholesterol levels also dropped 7 points—about 14 percent. The pressure-lowering chemical is called 3-n-butyl phthalide and gives celery its aroma.

Dr. Elliott says celery may be unique, because "the active blood pressure–lowering compound is found in rather high concentrations in celery, and not in many other vegetables." Dr. Elliott speculates that the celery lowers pressure by reducing blood concentrations of stress hormones that cause blood vessels to constrict. He suggests celery may be most effective in those whose blood pressure is linked to mental stress, which could be up to half of all Americans.

Note: Although celery is high in sodium compared with other vegetables, one medium stalk still contains a mere 35 milligrams of sodium. Thus, a two-stalk blood pressure–lowering dose would add only 70 daily milligrams of sodium, an insignificant amount in a total diet.

Garlic's Legendary Powers

Eat more garlic. It is another legendary folk remedy for high blood pressure, and it is effective, according to recent studies. Long used in China and widely used today in Germany as a blood pressure medication, garlic can have a striking impact.

An analysis of eight controlled studies found that taking 600 to 900 milligrams daily of Kwai, an over-the-counter garlic supplement (equal to one or two fresh garlic cloves), lowered mild blood pressure an average 8 percent in one to three months, according to Professors Christopher Silagy, University of South Australia, and Dr. Andrew Neil, Oxford University.

In a double-blind German test of Kwai, doses comparable to a couple of daily garlic cloves pushed diastolic blood pressure down in patients with mild high blood pressure. The blood pressure in the garlic group sank from an average 171/102 to 152/89 after three months, while the blood pressure of the placebo group stayed the same. Interestingly, garlic's impact grew stronger throughout the test, suggesting that daily infusions of garlic have a cumulative effect.

Garlic contains chemicals that act like ACE inhibitors, prescription drugs commonly given to lower blood pressure and protect the heart, according to Harry G. Preuss, M.D., of Georgetown University Medical School. In his tests of hypertensive rats, various types of garlic, including Kwai and Kyolic (another brand name supplement) significantly depressed blood pressure. Dr. Preuss says garlic also works by relaxing the smooth muscles of the blood vessels, allowing them to dilate, which is what happens in animals fed garlic juice. Both garlic and onions contain a great deal of a compound, adenosine, that is a smooth-muscle relaxant, according to George Washington University researchers. That means eating onions also should help reduce blood pressure. Additionally, onions contain small amounts of prostaglandin A1 and E, substances with blood pressure–lowering effect.

Note: Both raw and cooked garlic and onions can benefit blood pressure, although raw garlic is thought to be more potent.

Oh, for a Tin of Mackerel

Eat fatty fish. "My own blood pressure dropped from 140/90 to 100/70 after I started eating a small can of mackerel fillets every day," says researcher Peter Singer, Ph.D., of Berlin, Germany. Fish's main blood pressure medicine is thought to be omega-3 fatty acids in the oil. A string of studies on fish oil find it helps keep a lid on blood pressure. Dr. Singer, for example, found small doses of fish oil as effective in reducing blood pressure as the beta-blocker Inderal, a commonly prescribed blood pressure medication, as he reported at the 1990 International Conference on Fish Oils in Washington, D.C. He also found that Inderal and fish oil together reduced blood pressure better than either did alone. Thus, if just eating fish does not do the trick, it may still add to the potency of medication, making a lower dose possible.

How much fish is needed to lower blood pressure? University of Cincinnati tests found that blood pressure fell 4.4 points diastolic and 6.5 points systolic in subjects with mild blood pressure who took 2,000 milligrams of omega-3 fatty acids daily for three months. That's the amount in three and a half ounces of fresh Atlantic mackerel, four ounces of canned pink salmon, or seven ounces of canned sardines. The drop was enough to eliminate the need for medication in some people.

Another fascinating Danish study suggests that you need a minimum of three servings of fish a week to control blood pressure. Investigators found that adding fish oil to the diets of those who ate fish three or more times a week *did not reduce blood pressure further*. However, doses of fish oil did depress blood pressure in those who did not eat that much fish. Thus, it appears that fish eaten three times a week supplies enough omega-3 oil to control blood pressure in most people, which suggests high blood pressure is partly due to a "fish deficiency." Other components of seafood, such as potassium and selenium, may also contribute to lowering blood pressure.

- **BOTTOM LINE:** Eat fish at least three times a week, preferably fatty fish such as salmon, mackerel, herring, sardines, and tuna.

More Fruits and Vegetables

Medical fact: There's something magic about a fruit-and-vegetable-rich diet that curbs high blood pressure. Numerous studies point to fruits and vegetables as anti–high blood pressure agents. One of the most exciting recent studies, called DASH (Dietary Approaches to Stop Hypertension), showed that a diet rich in fruits and vegetables was, in many cases, as effective as medication in lowering blood pressure. In this eleven-week study, 459 people (133 of them with high blood pressure) ate four to five servings of fruits daily and four to five servings of vegetables, and kept the rest of the diet low in fat and rich in whole grains. In just two weeks, those with high blood pressure lowered their numbers by an average of 11.4 systolic and 5.5 diastolic (bottom number). That's about the same effect as drug therapy for mild hypertension, according to the study's authors. And, they estimate, adoption of this low-fat, fruit-and-vegetable-rich diet could "reduce the incidence of coronary heart disease by approximately 15 percent and stroke by approximately 27 percent." Interestingly, those with normal blood pressure also saw a little drop in their numbers, leading the researchers to speculate that this type of eating pattern also helps prevent high blood pressure.

There's good research backing up the prevention theory: A study looking at the eating habits of nearly 42,000 female nurses by Harvard researcher Alberto Ascherio showed that women who ate the most fruits and vegetables were least likely to have high blood pressure. The most protective: apples, oranges, prunes, grapes, carrots, alfalfa, mushrooms, raw spinach, and celery. And research regularly shows that vegetarians generally have lower blood pressure than meat eaters, and switching to a vegetarian diet can lower blood pressure.

Why are fruits and vegetables so powerful? Frank M. Sacks, M.D., an assistant professor of medicine at Harvard Medical School, says there are two obvious possibilities: something in plant foods depresses blood pressure or something in meat forces it up. At first Dr. Sacks thought meat raised blood pressure, but he scrapped the theory after he tested vegetarians by having them add meat to their diet. In one group of vegetarians who ate eight ounces of lean beef a day for a month, systolic blood pressure rose very slightly, diastolic blood pressure not at all. Neither did a heavy egg diet for three weeks boost blood pressure. Nor could he get blood pressure to budge in response to different kinds of fats. Dr. Sacks concluded that curbing total fat or saturated animal fat does not affect blood pressure at all.

On the other hand, he is convinced that agents in vegetables and fruits have mysterious powers to reduce blood pressure. One blood pressure–lowering drug may be fiber, especially from fruit. A Harvard study of nearly 31,000 middle-aged and elderly men found that those who ate very little fruit were 46 percent more likely to develop high blood pressure over the next four years than men who ate the fiber equivalent of five apples a day. For unknown reasons, fiber in fruit had the strongest antihypertensive effect, more so than fiber in vegetables or cereals.

Another possibility is antioxidants in fruits and vegetables that in roundabout fashion increase amounts of a hormone-like substance, prostacyclin, that dilates blood vessels and lowers pressure. Another explanation is vitamin C.

Vitamin C Up,
Blood Pressure Down

Eat vitamin C foods. A lack of vitamin C can send blood pressure up. In fact, vitamin C in fruits and vegetables is a powerful preventive medicine against high blood pressure, argues hypertension expert Dr. Christopher J. Bulpitt of the Hammersmith Hospital in London. He points to a string of evidence showing that high blood pressure and stroke fatalities are highest among people who eat the least vitamin C. Researcher Paul F. Jacques, at the U.S. Department of Agriculture's Human Nutrition Research Center on Aging at Tufts University, agrees that a low intake of foods rich in vitamin C predicts high blood pressure. In one study he found that elderly people who ate the vitamin C in a single orange a day were twice as likely to have high blood pressure as those who ate four times that much. Systolic pressure was 11 points higher and diastolic pressure 6 points higher among the skimpy vitamin C eaters. In other research, Dr. Jacques concluded that low blood levels of vitamin C raised systolic pressure about 16 percent and diastolic pressure 9 percent.

"There is something about not eating enough vitamin C that raises blood pressure," says Dr. Jacques. Thus, if you have high blood pressure, make sure you eat at least the vitamin C in an orange a day. There's also evidence that eating super amounts of vitamin C, in excess of correcting a deficiency, can further depress blood pressure. Dr. Jacques also stresses that other components in such fruits and vegetables besides vitamin C may help keep blood pressure in check. (For a list of foods rich in vitamin C, see the Appendix, pages 291–92)

Potassium Lowers Pressure

Don't neglect potassium, concentrated in fruits and vegetables and seafood. It, too, is strong hypertension medicine. There's no question that adding potassium to the diet can lower blood pressure and taking it away can raise it. In fact, deliberately eating a low-potassium diet can *cause* high blood pressure. As proof, in tests at Temple University School of Medicine, ten men with normal blood pressure ate a potassium-adequate diet, then a potassium-restricted diet, each for nine days. Deprived of potassium, the men experienced an average jump in arterial pressure (including both diastolic and systolic pressure) of 4.1 points—up from 90.9 to 95. Their blood pressure shot even higher when the men's diets were loaded with sodium. Thus, potassium also helps keep a high-sodium diet in check, said the study's senior author, G. Gopal Krishna, M.D. He theorizes that too little potassium leads to sodium retention, which over time may trigger high blood pressure.

Getting enough potassium can also lessen the doses of medication you need. A study at the University of Naples in Italy discovered that after a year on a high-potassium diet, 81 percent of a group of patients needed only half their original dosages of drugs to control their high blood pressure. Further, 38 percent of the high-potassium group was able to stop medication entirely. They simply ate three to six servings of high-potassium foods a day, boosting their average intake of potassium about 60 percent. (For a list of foods high in potassium, see pages 289–90.)

Go for Calcium-Rich Foods

A secret weapon against high blood pressure may be high-calcium foods. Some experts contend that high blood pressure is more likely due to a deficiency of calcium than to a surplus of sodium, and in fact, that adequate calcium can cancel the blood pressure–raising effects of sodium in some people. Of those Americans with mild to moderate hypertension, 20 to 40 percent would be able to either discontinue their antihypertensive medication or lower their dosages just by getting adequate calcium, according to Dr. David A. McCarron of Oregon Health Sciences University in Portland. Dr. McCarron says some individuals simply need more calcium than others to keep blood pressure normal, and quite often those are people who are "salt sensitive," that is, whose blood pressure rises from eating too much sodium. One theory is that such individuals retain water when they eat too much sodium, and that calcium acts like a natural diuretic to help kidneys release sodium and water, thus reducing blood pressure. Another, more complex, explanation is that calcium works by preventing release of the parathyroid hormone that can raise blood pressure.

Unquestionably, in some people calcium does reduce blood pressure. A recent study at Boston University found that men who ate the most calcium (322 to 1,118 milligrams daily) were 20 percent less apt to develop high blood pressure with age as men who ate the least calcium (8 to 109 mg daily). And research at the University of Texas Health Science Center showed that 800 milligrams of calcium a day reduced mild high blood pressure in 20 percent of subjects by a dramatic 20 to 30 points. Most, however, had small drops, and oddly, blood pressure went up in about 20 percent.

Another study found that people under age 40 may cut their chances of developing high blood pressure by eating enough calcium. In fact, the chances of high blood pressure went down an average 20 percent for each 1,000 milligrams of calcium consumed per day in moderate drinkers (not more than one drink a day) who were not overweight. The risk plunged by 40 percent in such people who drank less alcohol. Alcohol tends to counteract calcium's powers to lower blood pressure, said study author James H. Dwyer of the University of Southern California School of Medicine in Los Angeles. (For a list of high-calcium foods, see Appendix, page 288.)

Note: Milk and dairy foods, of course, are rich in calcium, and there's some evidence that drinking milk may help reduce blood pressure. However, since milk can cause digestive problems and allergies in many people, don't forget that many other foods are high in calcium—such as green leafy vegetables (kale, broccoli, collard greens, turnip greens) as well as canned sardines and salmon with bones.

Fiber Fix

Much research shows that high-fiber foods keep blood pressure down. A Harvard study found that women who ate 25 grams of fiber a day were 25 percent less apt to develop high blood pressure than those eating only 10 grams daily. Best bets are foods high in soluble type fiber, mainly fruits, vegetables, and rice and oats. Insoluble fibers, as in wheat bran, do not work as well. Dr. James Anderson, University of Kentucky, put diabetic men on a high soluble fiber diet and found that their blood pressure dropped 10 percent. (For a list of foods high in soluble fiber, see "Super Sources of Cholesterol-Fighting Fiber," pages 82-83.)

Try Olive Oil

Putting some olive oil in your diet may help lower blood pressure. A study by researchers at Stanford Medical School of seventy-six middle-aged men with high blood pressure a few years ago concluded that the amount of monounsaturated fat in three tablespoons of olive oil a day could lower systolic pressure about 9 points and diastolic pressure about 6 points. More remarkable, a University of Kentucky study found that a mere two-thirds of a tablespoon of olive oil daily reduced blood pressure by about 5 systolic points and 4 diastolic points in men. In a recent Dutch study, eating high amounts of olive oil drove down blood pressure slightly, even in those with normal pressure.

Further, a major analysis of the diets of nearly 5,000 Italians noted that those eating the most olive oil had lower blood pressure by 3 or 4 points, especially men. Among the Italians, those eating lots of butter had higher blood pressure.

To Salt or Not to Salt?

The first cure most people think of for high blood pressure is to cut down on salt. It may or may not work, depending on your individual biological make-up. Scientists have been arguing for years over the impact of salt on high blood pressure, and the debate goes on. It's unlikely that salt is a major *cause* of high blood pressure, concluded a recent Harvard report. Still, Dr. William Castelli, senior investigator of the famed Framingham Heart Study, notes that in the few areas of the world where salt intake is low, high blood pressure is rare and does not rise with age as it does among Americans. Also, if you have high blood pressure, restricting salt may help curb it, especially if you are among the one-third to one-half of those who are particularly sensitive to blood pressure boosts from sodium. Such "salt responders" are most apt to benefit from sodium cutbacks, say most experts. But you usually only know if you try it. There's even evidence that restricting sodium can depress normal blood pressure.

A major new study sponsored by the National Institutes of Health shows that for some people, cutting back on sodium means saying good riddance to blood pressure medication. The study, called TONE (Trial of Nonpharmacologic Interventions in the Elderly), looked at the effects of losing weight and/or reducing sodium on blood pressure on 875 men and women age 60 to 80, who were using medications to control their hypertension. Thirty-eight percent of those who reduced their daily sodium intake by about 900 milligrams were able to go off medication, and kept their blood pressure in check all thirty months of the research study.

How much improvement can you expect when you cut back on sodium? The University of London's Dr. Malcolm Law estimates that eliminating one teaspoon of salt (about 2,000 mg of sodium) a day from your diet can knock systolic pressure down an average 7 mmHg and diastolic down 3.5 mmHg if you have high blood pressure.

Restricting sodium may also give you younger blood vessels, which can help lower blood pressure, according to Ross D. Feldman of the University of Western Ontario. He and his colleagues noted that aging vessels lose some dilating ability, which may contribute to high blood pressure; sodium can aggravate the situation. In tests, Dr. Feldman's group found that cutting back on salt helped restore normal functioning in aged blood vessels. They showed that older people on a high-salt diet for four days had blood vessels that dilated only half as much as those of younger volunteers. But on a low-salt diet the older group's aged blood vessels dilated just as well as those of the younger group. This suggests, says Dr. Feldman, that a low-salt diet may be an antidote to declining blood vessel functions that raise blood pressure.

Note: One big way to cut down on sodium is to limit processed foods, which account for about 75 percent of the sodium in the food supply.

Sodium Surprise

Still, sodium restriction may not work for some people. In fact, in a small percentage of people, cutting down on sodium actually has the contrary action of driving blood pressure up, according to Dr. Bernard Lamport of the Albert Einstein College of Medicine. After reviewing the current research, he reported that from 20 to 25 percent of those with high blood pressure who moderately restrict their sodium intake, as many doctors recommend, have significant drops in blood pressure. On the other hand, blood pressure rises significantly in 15 percent of such patients. "In these people, salt restriction is hazardous," he insists.

As a test, Dr. Lamport advises people with high blood pressure to cut down on sodium for a couple of months under a doctor's supervision. If blood pressure goes down, fine, keep on; if it goes up, stop. But the point is, he emphasizes, everyone cannot count on sodium restriction to be a panacea for high blood pressure.

The National Institutes of Health advises everyone to eat no more than 6 grams of sodium a day—the amount in about three teaspoons of salt.

- **BOTTOM LINE:** Whether salt restriction controls your blood pressure depends on your individual biologic reaction. But even if you don't have high blood pressure, it's smart to go easy on salt because sodium may promote brain vessel damage and strokes in other ways than by boosting blood pressure, declares Louis Tobian Jr., M.D., hypertension chief at the University of Minnesota. And if you have kidney or heart problems in addition to high blood pressure, you most certainly should cut back on salt, he cautions.

How Sweet It Isn't

Sugar may be as big a villain in raising blood pressure as salt, warns Harry G. Preuss, M.D., of Georgetown University Medical School. And the American diet packed with both salt and sugar is worst of all, he says. In animal studies he finds that sugar and salt together boost blood pressure more than either alone. Sugar appears to disrupt the metabolism of insulin, a hormone that helps regulate blood pressure. Also, heavy sugar consumption induces salt and water retention. A possible way to blunt sugar-induced high blood pressure: take chromium supplements. They work in animals, says Dr. Preuss, who takes 500 micrograms of chromium daily. Other experts at the U.S. Department of Agriculture recommend 100 to 200 micrograms daily to help regulate insulin and blood sugar.

- **BOTTOM LINE:** Limit foods high in sugar and especially those foods high in both sodium and sugar, such as processed fruit pies and other snack foods.

Watch the Alcohol

Undeniably, alcohol can elevate blood pressure, according to overwhelming and consistent research. In both their 1992 and 1996 reviews of the evidence, physicians at the Royal Perth Hospital in Australia concluded that blood pressure goes up in men and women of all ethnic groups and ages in response to all varieties of alcoholic beverages, including beer, wine, and spirits. Further, the more you drink, the higher your blood pressure is expected to go, they found. Studies suggest that each daily drink drives systolic blood pressure up 1 mmHg, and that makes alcohol a greater blood pressure threat than sodium, according to the Australian experts.

In general, they reported that imbibing three or more drinks a day doubles the number of men and women who have high blood pressure of over 160/95.

"Three or more alcoholic drinks a day is the most common cause of reversible or curable hypertension."
—*N. M. Kaplan,*
University of Texas
Health Science Center, Dallas

A large-scale Harvard study of women nurses found that a couple of beers, two glasses of wine, or a shot of liquor a day had no effect on blood pressure. However, drinking more caused a steady, progressive rise in blood pressure. Compared to nondrinkers, women drinking between two and three drinks a day were 40 percent more likely to have elevated blood pressure. The risk was 90 percent greater in women drinking more than three drinks a day.

Blood pressure tends to drop when you cut back on alcohol. A study at Kaiser Permanente Hospital found that alcohol-associated high blood pressure dropped to normal within days after cutting out all booze. If you are a heavy drinker, some experts say, going on the wagon may bring blood pressure down as much as 25 points. Some reports show that heavy drinking or binge drinking—more than six drinks a day—may boost blood pressure by nearly 50 percent!

On the other hand, a little alcohol—less than one or two drinks daily—may somehow help keep blood pressure lower in moderate drinkers, compared with nondrinkers, finds Harvard's Matthew Gillman. Other research suggests red wine may be best. For instance, a large British study found that wine drinkers were less apt to have high blood pressure. The optimal amount appeared to be two or three glasses of red or white wine per week. In contrast, beer drinkers had higher blood pressure. In some studies, however, wine drinkers have better health habits than people who drink other types of alcohol, making it hard to tell if it's the wine or something else. Red wine's protective effect is probably due to chemicals, also found in purple grape juice, that tend to dilate and relax blood vessels, finds David F. Fitzpatrick at the University of South Florida College of Medicine.

He speculates such activity may reduce blood pressure and vascular spasms that can trigger heart attacks.

- **BOTTOM LINE:** How much can you safely drink without fear of raising blood pressure? No more than two drinks a day, according to the National Institutes of Health. Women shouldn't drink more than one drink a day; more may raise breast cancer risk. Also be aware that drinking alcohol can cancel out the benefits of both a low-sodium diet and blood pressure medication.

Few Worries About Coffee

Caffeine does not seem to be a prime culprit in chronic high blood pressure, say many researchers. Caffeine can temporarily raise blood pressure in occasional users, and even in regular caffeine users, particularly when they are under mental stress. But in the end, caffeine does not seem to have lasting effects on blood pressure or to shorten life in those with high blood pressure, insist researchers at the University of Texas Health Science Center. In a study of 10,064 Americans diagnosed with high blood pressure, the Texas team found that hypertensives who drank more tea or coffee—brewed, instant, or decaffeinated—were not more likely to die of heart disease or any other cause.

Nevertheless, if you are under mental stress, caffeine is more apt to drive up your blood pressure. For example, Dr. Joel Dimsdale of the University of California at San Diego had twelve healthy regular coffee drinkers solve arithmetic problems after they had drunk either regular or decaf coffee. In all cases, their blood pressure shot up more (an average 12 points systolic and 9 points diastolic) during the stressful tasks after they had consumed caffeine.

Additionally, the stress-caffeine combination may be more profound in those with high blood pressure or a genetic predisposition to it, according to Dr. Michael F. Wilson, a professor of medicine at the University of Oklahoma. He found that men at high risk of high blood pressure were much more apt to have blood pressure spurts when subjected to stress-producing tests after they had drunk the caffeine in two or three cups of coffee. Such people, when stressed, have an exaggerated adrenocortical response to caffeine that drives up blood pressure, he says.

- **BOTTOM LINE:** Most people with high blood pressure don't need to give up coffee. It usually does not push blood pressure into the "high zone" in healthy individuals, or aggravate it significantly in those who have high blood pressure. So concluded a special report on high blood pressure by the Harvard Health Letter. On the other hand, if you are commonly stressed-out, adding caffeine could be detrimental by helping boost blood pressure, say other experts.

Excess Pounds, Excess Blood Pressure

A major cause of high blood pressure is excessive weight. As much as one-third of high blood pressure sufferers are overweight. And losing weight is one of the surest ways to get your blood pressure down. That same TONE study that got the dramatic results from cutting back on salt also showed that moderate weight loss is very effective. In that study of 60- to 80-year-olds who had been controlling their blood pressure with medication for an average of eleven years, researchers helped overweight to very obese people lose an average of 9 pounds. After the weight loss, 37 percent didn't need the medication at all, and got a clean bill of cardiovascular health two years later. And a classic study published in the *New England Journal of Medicine* found that losing an average 23 pounds in two months depressed systolic pressure 26 points and diastolic 20 points. Blood pressure returned to normal in two-thirds of the patients. Every 1 mm drop in blood pressure translates to a 3 percent drop in heart disease risk; so the effects of weight loss can be tremendous.

Smaller weight losses also make a difference. In an experiment at the University of Texas Southwestern Medical Center in Dallas, people who lost 7 percent of their starting weight (on average, 15 pounds) lowered their blood pressure by an average of 12 points for systolic and 8 points for diastolic. "These results are to be expected when you lose that first 10 or 15 pounds; losing more probably won't bring blood pressure down much more," according to study leader Benjamin Levine, M.D., cardiologist and director of the university's Institute for Exercise and Environmental Medicine.

- **Bottom Line:** "If you have mild hypertension, try the diet and exercise route first. But if you have significant hypertension, get on medication first, then work on losing at least 10 pounds. When you've lost the weight, work with your doctor on seeing whether you can reduce the medication or stop taking it altogether," advises Dr. Levine.

Advice: Be sure before taking medication that your high blood pressure is properly diagnosed. New research shows that many people are diagnosed with chronic high blood pressure and medicated when in fact they have what is called "white coat hypertension," induced by stress or other factors when blood pressure is taken by a professional, notably in a doctor's office. Surest way to diagnose high blood pressure: attachment to a twenty-four-hour blood pressure monitoring device that takes and records blood pressure every half hour throughout an entire day. Consult your doctor about this. Next best way: taking your own blood pressure at home with a reliable monitor at different times of day.

Diet Prescription for High Blood Pressure

- The number one thing you can do is eat more fruits and vegetables of all kinds that are overflowing with known and unknown blood pressure–lowering agents, including vitamin C, potassium, and calcium. Vegetarians have strikingly low rates of high blood pressure.
- Especially eat garlic and celery.
- Fish is another must for the blood pressure–conscious. Its oil seems essential in keeping blood pressure on a healthful plateau. Eat fatty fish, such as mackerel, sardines, salmon, or herring, three times a week.
- Go easy on the salt shaker when cooking. And don't add salt at the table. Most of all, be wary of processed foods, which are often loaded with sodium. One study found that about 70 percent of all sodium in typical diets came from such processed foods.
- Keep your alcohol intake to a drink or two a day. And avoid binge drinking, which can drive your blood pressure up markedly.
- Don't consume caffeine excessively, especially if you are subject to high stress.
- If you are overweight, lose weight, which usually brings blood pressure down.

Part 2

What to Take to Overcome Heart Disease

The Frontier Beyond Food

Bothersome philosophical question: If we need heavy doses of vitamins and minerals, why didn't nature put them in food in the first place? Isn't it unnatural to take supra-natural doses in pills? No.

No matter how good your diet, the fact is, you must also take specific vitamin/mineral supplements to save yourself from atherosclerosis, heart attacks, and strokes as you get older. And if you have a heart attack, it's even more critical that you get the right therapeutic supplements to strengthen your heart and prevent future heart attacks and strokes.

The evidence is clear that such supplements can save you from becoming a victim of cardiovascular disease. Countless physicians, cardiologists, scientists, and researchers, who only a few years ago were skeptics, are now enthusiastically taking vitamin/mineral and herbal supplements and recommending them to patients. Fast disappearing is the dogma that food can give you everything you need to get through the tough years of old age and the looming specter of heart disease.

And if you do have symptoms of heart disease, including a heart attack or stroke, you may want to try tested nontraditional remedies instead of, or in addition to, mainstream pharmaceutical drugs. Such remedies are often much safer and can be equally effective or superior to prescription drugs.

Research has now progressed to the point that not taking supplements to save your heart is absolutely reckless.

What You Need to Know About Supplements to Fend Off Heart Disease

- Think of heart disease as partly a vitamin/mineral "deficiency disease" of global proportions.
- To best stave off heart disease, along with a nutrient-rich diet, it's necessary to take extra amounts of certain supplements, notably vitamin E, vitamin C, beta-carotene, and coenzyme Q-10.
- It's no longer smart to think that food can give you all the vitamins and minerals you need to fend off heart disease.
- You can't rely on the government-sanctioned recommended modest doses of vitamins and

minerals (RDAs and the like) to maximally combat heart disease, although sometimes even small amounts can reverse some risk factors for heart disease.

- Know that you are probably deficient even in the minimal recommended requirements for vitamins and minerals. Nearly all Americans are. Thus, you are flirting dangerously with heart disease.

- One of the main ways vitamins and minerals combat heart disease is by boosting antioxidant activity, helping crush free radicals that contribute to artery-clogging plaque and damaged vessels. Another way is by suppressing levels of homocysteine, an amino acid that is linked to heart disease.

- Contrary to what you sometimes hear, vitamins and minerals in heart disease–preventative doses are remarkably safe and free of side effects.

- Most supplements are cheap, especially compared with the enormity of good they do and the money they save in drugs, high-tech procedures, doctors' bills, and hospitalization.

- Numerous vitamins and minerals and phytochemicals work together to protect against heart disease. There is no one anti-heart disease miracle. A number of studies show that antioxidants work better in combination than individually.

Vitamins Are More Potent in Pills

Did you know: Vitamins taken as pills pack much more punch than vitamins consumed in food? That's because nutrients concentrated in pills are better absorbed. That means they have more *bioavailability*, or potency in the body. Recently an expert committee of the Institute of Medicine of the National Research Council determined that 0.5 (one-half) microgram (mcg) of folic acid in a supplement is about twice as active in the body as the identical 0.5 microgram taken in food. Thus, 400 micrograms of folic acid in a pill equals the activity of 800 mcg in food.

Agriculture researchers find that antioxidant carotenoids such as beta carotene and lutein are about four times more bioavailable when taken in pills than in food. Thus, experts say it takes only 1.5 milligrams (mg) of lutein in a pill to get the same obtained daily in foods, such as kale, spinach, and other leafy greens. Harvard research shows that people who ate foods with 6 mg of lutein daily cut their risk of macular degeneration, an age-related eye disease, by 43 percent.

This, of course, does not mean it's wise to depend on supplements and skimp on fruits and vegetables, which contain an array of beneficial chemicals, including dozens of vitamins, minerals, and fiber that provide protection against heart disease and premature aging. Countless studies show that fruits and vegetables dramatically cut the risk of heart disease and stroke.

But supplements are a vital part of preventing, treating, and even reversing heart disease.

Chapter 1

Vitamins E and C: Strong Heart Meds

They are the strongest, cheapest, safest heart medicine you can find; in fact it's risky not to take them.

There's compelling new evidence that vitamin C and vitamin E can open up diseased and clogged arteries so they dilate normally and blood flows through to feed heart cells. These vitamins can also dramatically help slow down, stop, and maybe even reverse atherosclerosis (hardening of the arteries) by acting as anti-inflammatory agents and fighting bad cholesterol and other artery-clogging substances. They may even have a direct impact on heart function. In some research the vitamins proved more potent against heart disease than pharmaceutical drugs.

What makes all this so exciting is the fact that these vitamins can rescue us even after our arteries have become diseased and clogged. Thus, we need not just sit around and do nothing, fearing the worst. The astonishing news is, if you can keep your arteries open despite the amount of plaque buildup, you are not apt to suffer a heart attack. And that's one thing these vitamins can do, according to new findings and a new understanding of the role of artery function in heart attacks. They offer hope to millions who are not nearly ill enough to consider taking risky pharmaceutical heart drugs. They also can intervene in serious heart failure. That's why many doctors now say that antioxidant vitamins C and E in particular have crossed the line from preventive to therapeutic, becoming a new heart medication that can help save you from cardiac disability and death.

Some researchers and doctors are now pioneering the use of antioxidant vitamins as adjunct therapy to stop the deterioration of arteries and even to restore heart function and clear arteries, with amazing success. We are entering a new age of the practice of "antioxidant medicine," says Balz Frei, Ph.D., a prominent antioxidant researcher at Boston University Medical Center. In some cases heart patients are simply taking vitamin supplements on their own, sometimes with astonishing results.

What Are They?

Vitamin C and vitamin E are potent antioxidants; this means they can block the destructive activity of chemicals in the body called oxygen free radicals. These free radicals are created internally by body metabolism and also enter the body through exposure to all kinds of chemicals, including air pollutants, cigarette smoke, fatty foods, and radiation. Free radicals attack cells, promoting malicious changes that underlie virtually every chronic disease. Free radicals are major culprits in heart disease; they promote buildup of plaque in arteries and abnormal vascular functions, such as dilation and contractions. Antioxidants block the deleterious activity of free radicals so they cannot destroy your arteries and heart.

National Institute on Aging researchers recently found that taking both vitamin C and vitamin E pills chopped death risk from any cause in half among 10,000 elderly persons ages 67 to 105. Further, the elderly vitamin takers had only one-third as many heart disease deaths as non-vitamin takers.

Vitamin E—What Is It?

Like all vitamins, E is essential, meaning our bodies can't manufacture it so we must get it from food (or supplements). Under the umbrella term "vitamin E" are an entire family of related compounds called tocopherols or tocotrienols. Of these, d-alpha-tocopherol is the most "biologically active," meaning it is the most potent and the most efficient at performing its important functions. E is a fat-soluble vitamin, meaning that it's chemically comfortable attaching itself to fat. That's why E is found in vegetable oils, nuts, avocados, and other high-fat foods. We absorb fat-soluble vitamins along with fatty foods, so it's best to take vitamin E along with a meal containing at least a little fat.

The Evidence

Zaps Heart Attacks: For decades studies have linked increased vitamin E intake with less heart disease. Then in 1993 two compelling Harvard studies shocked the medical community into paying attention. Both studies showed that taking vitamin E supplements seemed to drastically reduce the appearance of heart disease. First in women: Among 87,000 nurses, incidence of major heart disease was 41 percent lower in those who reported taking from 100 to 250 IU daily of vitamin E pills for more than two years compared with those who did not take vitamin E supplements. Such vitamin takers also had a 29 percent lower stroke risk and a decrease in overall mortality rates of 13 percent.

Men were saved, too. Among 40,000 middle-aged men, those taking more than 100 IU of vitamin E a day for more than two years showed a 37 percent lower risk of major cardiovascular mishaps, including heart attacks. Vitamin E does not work overnight. The Harvard research suggests you must take vitamin E for at least two years before heart attack protection kicks in.

Important fact: Harvard authors Meir J. Stampfer, M.D., and Eric B. Rimm, Sc.D., stressed that you can't get enough vitamin E in food to suppress heart attacks. That requires vitamin E supplements, which both authors take. However, more than 250 IU a day did not additionally cut heart disease in their study.

Question: Can you afford *not* to take vitamin E?

Answer: The penalty may be harsh, if the Harvard study is accurate. "The risk for not taking vitamin E was equivalent to the risk of smoking," marveled Dr. Rimm.

In fact, the study indicated that the benefits of taking vitamin E far exceeded the benefits seen from reducing high blood pressure and high cholesterol! A large World Health Organization study of men in sixteen European cities agreed that high blood levels of vitamin E are more apt to prevent fatal heart attacks than lowering blood cholesterol is.

In 1996 along came a blockbuster study from the University of Cambridge in England that showed without a doubt how powerful vitamin E supplements are, not just in preventing heart disease, but remarkably, in treating it! The study by Professor Morris Brown and Dr. Malcolm Michinson was conducted on 2,000 people with confirmed artery disease, including a history of heart attack. Over the next eighteen months, half the heart disease patients took a single daily dose of either 400 IU or 800 IU of natural vitamin E; the others took a placebo (dummy pill). The results were so amazing that even the investigators were surprised. The users of either dose of vitamin E suffered only 23 percent as many nonfatal heart attacks as those taking the placebo. Vitamin E had slashed the incidence of heart attacks by an astounding 77 percent. The researchers pronounced vitamin E more powerful in controlling heart attacks than aspirin or cholesterol-lowering drugs. Indeed, they found that vitamin E reduced the risk of nonfatal heart attack to normal—that expected in healthy individuals with no signs of heart disease. Further, the benefits of the vitamin-drug were evident within six and a half months after subjects started to take it.

Unclogs Arteries: Studies in monkeys, our closest relatives, have found that clogging of arteries induced by a high-fat diet is prevented and reversed by modest doses of vitamin E. In a remarkable six-year research project, Anthony J. Verlangieri, Ph.D., of the University of Mississippi's Atherosclerosis Research Laboratory fed monkeys a high-fat lard-cholesterol diet. Naturally, their arteries became clogged and blocked, but when the monkeys also got vitamin E, the extent of artery blockage dropped 60 to 80 percent. More spectacular, feeding the monkeys a daily dose of 108 international units (IU) of vitamin E *after* their arteries were seriously clogged cleared the artery blockage by about 60 percent. The blockages shrank from an average 35 percent artery closure to a 15 percent closure in two years!

Taking vitamin E supplements also can retard artery clogging and open up arteries in humans. Dr. Howard N. Hodis at the University of Southern California School of Medicine found that men who said they took 100 IU or more of vitamin E daily after coronary bypass surgery had less-narrowed arteries after two years than non-vitamin users or those taking lower doses of vitamin E. Furthermore, angiograms (X-rays) showed clearly that the plaque in the arteries of some of the vitamin E takers had shrunk, signifying a retreat or regression in atherosclerosis.

How Does It Work?

The main way vitamin E fights heart disease is probably by its profound effects on blood cholesterol. It does not necessarily lower cholesterol, but it helps stop bad LDL cholesterol from being chemically changed, a process that promotes cholesterol's ability to infiltrate artery walls, creating destructive plaque. Vitamin E enters the LDL cholesterol molecule and inhibits hazardous oxidation (rancidity), thus switching off the very genesis of coronary heart disease. A study by Ishwarlal Jialal of the University of Texas Southwestern Medical Center in Dallas found that taking 800 IU of vitamin E a day for three months slashed LDL cholesterol oxidation—and thus its ability to foster artery damage and heart disease—a dramatic 40 percent! "It's very clear that vitamin E is the most potent antioxidant against LDL oxidation," he says. He found it takes at least 400 IU of vitamin E per day to significantly prevent LDL cholesterol from being oxidized. Studies in animals and humans consistently show that a daily dose of 400 to 500 IU of vitamin E drastically inhibits the propensity of LDL to become toxic and damage arteries. Studies show that vitamin E also can slow down the proliferation of smooth muscle cells that pile up on artery walls, contributing to artery-clogging plaque.

Researchers at the University of Bern in Switzerland have discovered another way vitamin E discourages artery clogging. The vitamin keeps arteries open by inhibiting the proliferation of smooth muscle cells that contributes to clogged arteries. The Swiss researchers demonstrated that rabbits given vitamin E had only half as much damage to the aortas of their hearts as rabbits not given vitamin E. Indeed, vitamin E both prevented the occurrence of so-called fatty streaks, the earliest sign of artery damage—and kept artery damage from progressing once it occurred later in life. Thus, it's clear that plenty of vitamin E, which you can get only from supplements, is needed both early and throughout life to keep arteries open and flexible.

"Anyone with a family history of heart disease would be foolish not to take daily vitamin E supplements."
—*Ishwarlal Jialal, M.D., associate professor of internal medicine, the University of Texas Southwestern Medical Center at Dallas, and a leading researcher on vitamin E*

How Much? Dr. Jialal finds that 400 IU daily of vitamin E are required to help defuse bad type LDL cholesterol, thwarting its ability to clog arteries. Also, in the Cambridge study, 400 IU was as good as 800 IU in deterring heart attacks. Among researchers and doctors, the typical daily supplement dose of vitamin E is 400 IU. That dose also boosts immunity, according to research at Tufts University.

Safety: Most experts consider daily doses of 400 to

800 IU very safe, with no known toxic effects. Indeed, a one-year study of 800 patients found no adverse effects from a daily dose of 2,000 IU of vitamin E. In doses exceeding 400 IU, however, vitamin E, like aspirin, does have mild anticlotting activity, "thinning the blood," and is not recommended for people taking anti-coagulant drugs or facing surgery. Toxicity can occur at over 3,200 IU daily; signs include headaches, diarrhea, and elevated blood pressure. "Don't take more than 1,000 IU daily," advises Dr. Jialal.

In a recent Finnish study, vitamin E may have contributed to hemorrhagic or "bleeding stroke" in smokers, although most experts believe that the 50 IU dose used was too low to alter blood coagulation or to have other beneficial or detrimental effects.

Dr. Andreas Papas, a vitamin E expert at Eastman Kodak Company, notes that certain individuals seem to have an unusual sensitivity to vitamin E, causing blood pressure to rise. His advice: If you are concerned, stop taking vitamin E and see if blood pressure falls. Also, if you suspect a sensitivity to vitamin E, try mixed tocopherols rather than plain alpha-tocopherol. A mixture of various tocopherols (another name for vitamin E) is less apt to boost blood pressure, he speculates.

Caution: If you are taking anticoagulants, or suspect any type of bleeding problem, check with your doctor before taking vitamin E. It can have an anticoagulant effect.

False Alarm: Recent media reports suggested that a study at the University of California at Berkeley

showed that the most common type vitamin E supplement—alpha tocopherol—could be dangerous.
But scientists who did the study say that is not what
they found. "We were misquoted," says lead researcher
Dr. Bruce Ames. The study merely showed that a different form of vitamin E, gamma-tocopherol, also has
health merit as an antioxidant and might be added to
supplements to make them even better. "We are not
advocating that people stop taking vitamin E," he
says. Nearly all studies showing benefits of vitamin E,
including those reported in this book, have used common alpha-tocopherol supplements and not gamma or
mixed tocopherols.

What Kind? Vitamin E supplements are sold as synthetic (dl-alpha-tocopherol) or natural (d-alpha tocopherol), as noted on labels. Both have helped block
dangerous artery-clogging changes in bad LDL cholesterol in various studies, but natural is superior, according
to a review of thirty studies by Robert V. Acuff, Ph.D.,
a leading vitamin E authority at East Tennessee State
University. Apparently, the human body prefers natural vitamin E; it's better absorbed and is retained
longer in tissues than the synthetic type.

"Natural vitamin E may cost twice as much, but you
get twice as much bang for your buck," agrees Dr.
Graham W. Burton at the National Research Council
of Canada in Ottawa. Burton's recent study found that
doses of natural vitamin E boosts blood and organ levels of the antioxidant twice as high as does synthetic
vitamin E. Natural E was used in the highly successful
Cambridge heart study.

Pills vs. Food: This is one nutrient that you absolutely must supplement with to get therapeutic doses. Vitamin E is found primarily in fatty foods, which many Americans now restrict. Best sources: vegetable and seed oils. Good sources: sunflower seeds, almonds, wheat germ, filberts, peanuts, avocados, fortified cereals. To get 400 IU vitamin in food, you would have to eat about 20,000 calories a day, most in fat, say experts.

Is Your Heart Worth It?

Critics who call vitamins a waste of money are way off base. Actually, for every dollar spent on vitamin E, we save $50 in the cost of heart disease, figures Daniel Dranove, Ph.D., professor of Health Sciences at Northwestern University. His reasoning: Medical expenses and lost productivity from heart disease cost $200 billion yearly. Regularly taking vitamin E can cut heart disease at least 20 percent, research indicates. That gives vitamin E "a benefit-to-cost ratio of 50 percent or more," he concludes.

Vitamin C—What Is It?

Like vitamin E and all vitamins, vitamin C is essential because we need it to survive; our bodies cannot manufacture it, and we must get it through diet or supplements. Its chemical name is ascorbic acid. For years sailors knew that eating citrus fruit prevented the dreaded disease scurvy. Finally in 1932 a University of Pittsburgh scientist pinpointed the anti-scurvy compound as vitamin C.

The Alarming Facts

- One-fourth of Americans do not get even the minimal rock-bottom amount of 60 milligrams of vitamin C that cells need to perform basic biological functions.
- Only 9 percent of Americans eat five daily fruits and vegetables (200 to 300 milligrams of vitamin C) urged by the National Cancer Institute.
- About 20 percent of healthy older people and 68 percent of elderly nonhospitalized patients had white blood cells deficient in vitamin C, according to one study.

The Evidence

You've heard that vitamin C may fight colds. Well, that's nothing compared with what scientists say it may actually do—help stop our epidemic of heart disease, and other chronic diseases. Vitamin C does more than fight free radical damage to LDLs; it offers wholesale protection of arteries. Modest amounts of vitamin C can drive up good type HDL cholesterol that discourages artery clogging, lower high blood pressure, strengthen blood vessel walls, make blood less sticky, and thwart cholesterol-inspired changes leading to clogged arteries. Vitamin C is a potent water-soluble antioxidant that traps and disarms free radicals in the watery part of tissues. It also regenerates exhausted vitamin E and all-important glutathione, and spurs enzymes to search and destroy free radicals. Thus, for optimal aging slowdown, it's critical that cells have enough of both antioxidants E and C.

Saves Arteries: In one recent test of forty-six patients with coronary heart disease documented by angiogram, Boston University's Dr. Balz Frei and colleagues Joseph A. Vita and John Keaney Jr. reversed the dysfunctional way arteries relaxed by giving patients a dose of 2,000 milligrams of vitamin C. Ultrasound clearly showed that two hours after taking vitamin C, dilation of an artery in the arm improved by 50 percent in most patients and even more in those with the greatest initial vascular dysfunction. Indeed, after they took vitamin C the vascular function of the arteries in patients with heart disease was perfectly normal, dramatically reducing chances that the artery would malfunction, triggering a heart attack. Vitamin C, the researchers suggest, works primarily as an antioxidant to zap free radicals that otherwise suppress activity of nitric oxide needed to keep arteries properly relaxed. Lower doses may have a similar benefit, says researcher Balz Frei.

Further, 600 and 1,000 milligrams of vitamin C daily lessened heart damage and irregular heartbeats in patients, according to other new research.

Harvard researchers have shown that infusing vitamin C directly in the arteries of the heart also corrects vascular impairment in diabetics, which is similar to that in heart patients.

In another landmark study, vitamin C was successfully used as a post-angioplasty drug to keep arteries open, according to Japanese cardiologists at the Tokai University in Kanagawa. Angioplasty is a procedure often used to unblock clogged arteries. Because the arteries frequently close up again within several months, doctors are always looking for ways to prevent this reclosure. In the new Japanese study of 119 patients, a daily dose of 500 milligrams of vitamin C was incredibly effective. Four months after the surgery only 24 percent of those who took vitamin C had reclosed arteries—or restenosis, as it is called—compared with 43 percent of the patients who did not get vitamin C.

By anybody's standards it was a blockbuster result. A modest dose of an absolutely safe pill costing a few cents a day nearly *doubled* the chances of a successful heart procedure. Further, it reduced the need for repeat surgery by about 60 percent. Only 12 percent of those who took vitamin C needed another heart procedure, compared with 29 percent of those who were not getting vitamin C. Harvard professor Thomas Graboys, director of the Lown Cardiovascular Center at Brigham and Women's Hospital in Boston, agrees that vitamin C "can't hurt and may help" in treating people with heart disease.

Vitamins Vanquish McDonald's

One of the most fascinating research projects pitted vitamin C and vitamin E against the high-fat fare of McDonald's. It was done by researchers at the University of Maryland and showed that vitamin C and vitamin E help counteract the ill effects of eating lots of fast-food fat by preserving good vascular functioning. Twenty faculty members, supervised by cardiologist Gary Plotnik, each ate a 50 percent fat, 900 calorie breakfast at McDonald's, consisting of one Egg McMuffin, one Sausage McMuffin, and two servings of hash browns. Using ultrasound, the researchers scanned the main artery of their arms. As expected, the fat burden caused their arteries to dilate abnormally, so blood flow was sluggish.

On another day the same subjects ate the same breakfast, except that this time, about fifteen minutes before pigging out, they took 1,000 milligrams of vitamin C and 800 IU of vitamin E. The results were astounding. The ultrasound showed that despite the fat overload, the subjects' arteries continued to dilate normally, allowing a normal blood flow to feed the heart muscle. Indeed, the vitamins reversed a major ill effect of the high-fat breakfast that otherwise could trigger heart attack. The benefits lasted for six hours. This confirms the mounting evidence that vitamin C as well as vitamin E are potent medicines for regulating artery functions.

Brings Down Blood Pressure: Much research suggests that vitamin C can both prevent and reduce high blood pressure. Tufts University researchers found that people failing to get the daily vitamin C in an orange (70 milligrams) had 11 points higher systolic (upper number) and 6 points higher diastolic (lower number) pressure than those who ate more vitamin C. Consistently, people with high blood levels of vitamin C have lower blood pressure, according to research by Elaine B. Feldman, Medical College of Georgia. She also found that taking 1,000 milligrams of vitamin C daily lowered normal blood pressure about 4 percent. "Vitamin C seems to have unique pharmacological activity," she said. A gram of vitamin C can also lower blood pressure, according to U.S. Department of Agriculture studies. Among people with high blood pressure, a daily 1,000 milligram dose of vitamin C reduced both systolic and diastolic pressure about 7 percent.

How Does It Work?

As it turns out, vitamin C does lots more than prevent scurvy. Acting as an antioxidant, it protects arteries by neutralizing bad LDL cholesterol. Vitamin C is also a powerful vasodilator, and that is probably its more important method of fighting heart disease. This miraculous heart drug works by activating or releasing the chemical nitric oxide in artery walls. Nitric oxide, according to a rush of new research, is an amazing chemical. It controls the relaxation and constriction of arteries that maintain or cut off blood flow to the heart and brain. Moreover, nitric oxide inhibits the proliferation of smooth muscle cells that accumulate to build up the mass known as atherosclerotic plaque. Thus, indirectly through manipulating nitric oxide, vitamin C influences artery health.

However, vitamin C does even more. Blood clots tend to form on artery walls where a bit of plaque ruptures because it is weak and unstable. Scientists now realize that it is not primarily the *amount* of plaque lining your artery walls that creates heart attacks, but the *stability* of the plaque. If the composition of the plaque is stronger and less apt to rupture, clots and heart attacks are less apt to ensue. And what makes plaque more stable? Vitamin C, by spurring production and repair of collagen, a kind of cement that keeps plaque from fragmenting and creating hazardous blood clots.

How Much? Generally, research shows that you need from 500 to 1,000 milligrams of vitamin C daily. Smokers need at least twice as much as nonsmokers, because their bodies use up gobs of vitamin C trying to combat free radicals in smoke. Smokers consistently have low blood levels of vitamin C. So do "passive smokers," who inhale secondhand smoke.

Safety: Vitamin C is very safe, although taking too much typically causes diarrhea, possibly nausea and heartburn in some persons. A "bowel tolerance" dose is highly individualistic and usually requires more than 1,000 milligrams a day, more if you are ill. No serious adverse effects were reported in eight recent studies from taking up to 10,000 milligrams of vitamin C daily for several years. There's no evidence vitamin

C causes kidney stones. Nor do high doses of vitamin C cause "iron overload"—the harmful accumulation of iron in the body—in normal people, according to a review of research by the late Charles E. Butterworth, M.D., emeritus professor at the University of Alabama at Birmingham. Vitamin C supplements can exacerbate iron toxicity in those with genetic disorders in handling iron, notably a condition called hemochromatosis. Such persons should consult a physician before taking vitamin C supplements.

What Type? Vitamin C of any type appears to work. The type effective in Dr. Frei's artery study was a low-cost brand from a drugstore. Some experts favor a more expensive vitamin C called Ester-C, claiming it has more antioxidant power.

How Often? To keep your cells on total antioxidant alert with vitamin C, take your supplement quota three or four times a day rather than in one big dose. Throwing down a couple of 500 milligram pills at one time, particularly in the morning, instead of taking them throughout the day cheats your cells, because much of it is excreted in your urine. The body eliminates even large doses in twelve hours, and time-release doses in sixteen hours. The only way to keep levels of vitamin C continuously up in your blood is to take 500 milligrams every twelve hours, says Alfred B. Ordman, biochemistry professor at Beloit College in Beloit, Wisconsin.

Pills vs. Foods: Vitamin C, unlike vitamin E, is plentiful in the food supply. But unlike our Stone Age forefathers, who ate a hefty 400 milligrams of vitamin

C a day (about half a dozen oranges) by foraging for fruit and wild greens, most of us don't come close. So if you eat lots of vitamin C–rich fruits and vegetables (at least five servings a day), you can get fairly high doses of the vitamin, enough to discourage certain chronic diseases, such as cataracts and cancer. But to be safe, take a vitamin supplement in addition to, not as a substitute for, fruits and vegetables. (Remember, fruits and vegetables are packed with other antioxidants essential to postponing disease.) Foods high in vitamin C are sweet peppers, cantaloupe, pimentos, papaya, strawberries, Brussels sprouts, citrus fruits and juices, kiwi fruit, broccoli, tomatoes and tomato juice.

Chapter 2

Beta Carotene:
The Real Heart Story

Beta carotene is good for your heart—whether you get it in food or pills. But a major question seems to be, how much is needed in supplements and how much is safe for most people?

The Evidence

Saves Arteries: In a large Harvard study of 22,000 male physicians, investigators found no evidence that beta carotene supplements generally reduced the risk of heart disease. But the story was quite different in a group of about 300 doctors in the study who already had cardiovascular trouble or had suffered a heart attack. Taking 50 milligrams of beta carotene every other day for twelve years did reduce their risk of fatal heart attacks, strokes, and heart disease incidence by 33 percent compared with those taking a dummy pill. According to Charles Hennekens, M.D., head of the Harvard study, protection kicked in after two years, suggesting that beta carotene slows the progression of plaque buildup in arteries. He speculates that beta carotene supplements may be most beneficial to those already weakened by heart disease.

Why beta carotene supplements did not have a bigger impact on the Harvard physicians in general is not known. One possibility, according to Dr. Hennekens, is that beta carotene may not work best as an antioxidant alone, but in cooperation with other artery-protecting antioxidants, such as vitamins E and C. Indeed, studies have shown that all three have greater antioxidant impact than any one alone. Further, some say the synthetic form of beta carotene used in the study is not as protective as natural beta carotene.

How Does It Work?

There's compelling evidence beta carotene acts as an antioxidant to help defuse the dangers of bad LDL cholesterol, thus the destruction of arteries. A new study by Dr. Andrew J. Clifford at the University of California at Davis confirms that beta carotene supplements help block hazardous oxidation of LDL cholesterol, lessening cholesterol's ability to clog arteries. Dr. Clifford found that only 5.37 milligrams a day of natural beta carotene in supplements protected LDL.

How Much? As insurance against heart disease, some experts recommend 10 to 15 milligrams of beta carotene a day for nonsmokers. But as Dr. Clifford's study shows, only 6 milligrams daily in a supplement may be enough for most people. Some authorities advise current smokers not to take any beta carotene supplements or to limit such supplements to 8 to 10 milligrams a day.

Safety: Beta carotene is considered one of the most nontoxic of supplements. Studies in Italy, for example, using 90 milligrams of beta carotene daily have shown no significant signs of toxicity. Hundreds of studies on laboratory animals using very high doses of beta carotene have detected virtually no toxicity. High doses, however, can cause yellowing of skin, which disappears when you cut back on beta carotene.

Caution: Don't confuse beta carotene with plain retinol type vitamin A, which is derived from animal foods, such as liver, and can build up to toxic levels in your liver. Many multivitamin preparations contain high amounts of such retinol vitamin A. Adults should not take more than 5,000 to 10,000 IU of plain retinol vitamin A daily except on a physician's advice.

Pills vs. Food: You can get lots of beta carotene in fruits and vegetables, although the beta carotene in supplements is better absorbed, according to tests at the U.S. Department of Agriculture. Your body can also absorb more beta carotene from vegetables, such as carrots, that are lightly cooked. Heavy cooking destroys beta carotene.

What About the Cancer Scare?

Several years ago two studies—one in Finland, the other at the University of Washington—both suggested that high doses of beta carotene might promote lung cancer in some people. Unfortunately, the headlines were all that many people noticed or remembered. But the headlines did not tell the whole story. The facts are more enlightening and less frightening: Beta carotene did appear to raise the risk of developing lung cancer by about 20 percent in current, usually longtime heavy smokers. It is suspected that such victims may already have had undetected early signs of lung cancer.

In contrast, those who had quit smoking and took the beta carotene supplements actually were protected; they had a reduced lung cancer risk of 20 percent. In the Harvard study, the large doses of beta carotene also reduced the risk of prostate cancer by 36 percent in the subgroup of 300 physicians. Thus, it appears that the danger of beta carotene supplements applies entirely to current smokers, especially to smokers who also drink alcohol heavily.

Recently Tufts University researchers discovered a probable reason for beta carotene's increased threat to smokers. They sudied ferrets, animals that metabolize beta carotene the same way as humans.

The animals got the human daily equivalent of 30 milligrams of beta carotene. Some of the beta carotene was converted to an anticancer compound, but the excess beta carotene was stored and oxidized by high oxygen levels in lung cells, a process that promotes cell division and cancer. When the oxidizing effects of cigarette smoke on lung cells are added, the chances of cancer skyrocket, said researchers.

The message: A little beta carotene can retard cancer; too much may promote cancer in smokers. The safe anticancer dose for smokers, said Tufts biochemist Xiang-Dong Wang, is 8 to 10 milligrams of beta carotene. "Beta carotene gotten from fruits and vegetables is completely safe," he added.

The Triple Antioxidant Hit

You can get heart help from any one of the three antioxidant staples: vitamin E, vitamin C, and beta carotene. Each individually packs plenty of antioxidant power at fighting off bodily deterioration due to free radicals. But the three together are even more impressive. For example, here's what Harvard researchers found in epidemiological studies of 87,000 female nurses. In women getting lots of vitamin E, mostly from supplements (more than 200 IU daily), the odds of major cardiovascular disease dropped 34 percent. High intakes of beta carotene slashed heart disease risk 22 percent. High vitamin C intake reduced the odds 20 percent. But in women getting the highest amounts of all three antioxidants, heart disease risk dropped nearly 50 percent!

For one thing, the three antioxidants work together to inhibit the oxidation of bad LDL cholesterol leading to plaque buildup in arteries. In a recent Australian study, researchers gave subjects daily doses of 900 milligrams of vitamin C, 200 milligrams of vitamin E, and 18 milligrams of beta carotene. The result: The vitamins delayed the onset of oxidation of

LDL cholesterol by 28 percent after three months. After six months, the antioxidation effect was even stronger.

Most remarkable, the three vitamins worked in sequence and in complementary fashion to delay LDL oxidation. When vitamin E was exhausted, beta carotene took over. However, if enough vitamin C was present, it regenerated vitamin E's powers. Thus, the three antioxidants together seem most effective at reducing the danger of LDL oxidation.

Eating more antioxidants throughout your life can also help defeat rising blood pressure as you age. In one study, noted authority Jeremiah Stamler of Northwestern University Medical School in Chicago found that the blood pressure of men who ate the most vitamin C and beta carotene over ten years did not rise as much as that of those eating the least of such vitamins. The difference, though small, translates into a 6 percent reduction in deaths from stroke, 4 percent from heart disease, and 3 percent from all causes.

Chapter 3

B Vitamins Battle Heart Disease

Scientists have discovered another enemy of the heart—homocysteine—but fortunately they've also discovered a weapon to fight this enemy: B vitamins.

B vitamins have jumped to the forefront in fighting heart disease because of new discoveries about a villainous amino acid in the blood called homocysteine. If not properly metabolized, homocysteine interacts with bad LDL cholesterol to clog arteries. Homocysteine also make blood stickier and more prone to form blood clots. For thirty years medicine ignored the theory that vitamin B deficiencies triggered heart disease and strokes. Now strong evidence finds that three B vitamins can save arteries. Essential in disposing of homocysteine are three enzymes derived from vitamins B6, B12, and folic acid (folic acid is considered the most important). Consequently, a deficiency of these critical B vitamins allows homocysteine to build up in the blood, destroying arteries, promoting heart attacks, strokes, and deaths.

The Evidence

The evidence is steadily coming in showing that supplementing with B vitamins not only lowers homocysteine, but reduces other heart-risky conditions. How destructive is homocysteine? Experts report high homocysteine can boost the risk of vascular disease as much as fivefold, and heart disease deaths sixfold. Harvard researcher Meir Stampfer estimated that at least 150,000 of all heart attacks yearly are tied to high homocysteine levels. In a five-year Norwegian study of about 900 patients, those with high homocysteine blood levels had about six times the death rates as those with low homocysteine. Even when artery damage was not severe, high homocysteine seemed to help trigger heart attacks, the analysis showed.

Yet, high homocysteine is virtually cured by safe, inexpensive doses of three B vitamins—folic acid, B6, and B12. Reducing high homocysteine may have the same impact in fighting heart disease as lowering blood cholesterol from 275 to 189, says University of Michigan's Dr. Gilbert S. Omenn.

Quashes Homocysteine: Taking only 400 micrograms daily of a folic acid supplement controls homocysteine in most people, according to new tests by M. Rene Malinow at Oregon Health Sciences University. He says 400 micrograms work as well as 1,000 or 2,000 micrograms. University of Washington researchers recently concluded that inadequate folic acid causes 56,000 heart disease deaths yearly.

A new study that recruited men and women from nine European countries supports the B vitamin/homocysteine link. The study compared 750 people with heart disease to 800 people free of heart disease. Homocysteine levels, and blood levels of folate, B6, and B12 were measured. As you might expect, those with heart disease had higher levels of homocysteine, and as a rule had lower blood levels of folic acid and B6. In fact, 35 percent of heart disease victims were clinically B6 deficient.

The study revealed something extra heart-helpful about B6. The more B6 in the blood, the lower the risk for heart disease. Yes, B6 helps suppress homocysteine, but that is not the whole explanation, says lead researcher Killian Robinson. Even when homocysteine was normal, a B6 deficiency predicted blocked blood vessels in the heart, brain, and leg, he found. So regardless of homocysteine levels, a blood deficiency of B6 was still "a very powerful risk factor for heart disease and stroke," according to Dr. Robinson. He believes vitamin B6 apparently protects arteries in other ways, perhaps by deterring blood clots and altering cholesterol. Animals fed a diet deficient in B6 develop heart disease. Dr. Robinson says about 20 percent of Americans have a B6 deficiency, which "marks" them as heart disease targets.

Curbs Cardiovascular Disease: A University of Minnesota study lends more weight to the theory that B6 is uniquely heart-protective. The study, headed by Aaron Folsom, M.D., of 759 middle-aged men and women, identifies B6 as a primary predictor of heart disease. The researchers analyzed subjects' blood samples in 1987, then tracked the subjects for eight years. During that time, those with the highest blood levels of B6 had about one-third the chances of developing heart disease as those with the lowest B6 levels.

And a new fourteen-year Harvard study of 80,000 women nurses found that women who took in the most vitamin B6 and folic acid were about a third less likely to develop heart disease as those getting the least B vitamins. For maximum protection, Harvard researchers concluded, women must get a daily total from food and supplements of at least 400 micrograms (mcg) folic acid and 3 milligrams (mg) vitamin B6. In this study the most was 696 mcg of folic acid and 4.8 mg of B6 daily; the least was 158 mcg of folic acid and 1.1 mg of B6.

These findings are consistent with studies showing that people with heart disease have lower blood levels of folic acid and B6 than those free of heart disease, and with other research showing that supplementing with the three Bs lowers blood homocysteine levels.

Artery Scrubber: Folic acid and vitamin B6, and to a lesser extent vitamin B12, help suppress homocysteine. A new groundbreaking study by Canadian cardiologist J. David Spence, M.D., in the British medical journal *The Lancet*, offers the first evidence that lowering homocysteine with B vitamins profoundly benefits arteries. He and colleagues measured the progressive closure and plaque buildup in the carotid neck arteries of thirty-eight men and women, average age 58, before and after taking B vitamins for four and a half years. The daily doses: 2.5 mg folic acid, 250 micrograms B12, and 25 mg B6.

When the subjects were not taking B vitamins, their plaque area increased about 50 percent. After they took vitamins, the plaque actually decreased in size about 10 percent. In short, the vitamins helped clean out arteries and reverse atherosclerosis.

Beyond Homocysteine—Stroke Stopper: The Bs may also help save you from a first or second stroke. In a recent study of fifty stroke victims, half got B vitamins for three months, half didn't. The B group took in 5 milligrams (500 micrograms) of folic acid, 100 milligrams of vitamin B6, and 1 milligram (1,000 micrograms) of vitamin B12. At the study's end, homocysteine levels plunged in the B group and so did levels of thrombomodulin, a substance that circulates in the blood, signaling damage to the inner lining of blood vessels (called the endothelial cell lining). Nothing changed in the group that didn't receive the vitamins. "A lower level of thrombomodulin following high dose B vitamin therapy to lower homocysteine suggests reduced damage to the lining of the arteries," said lead researcher Richard F. Macko, M.D., associate professor of neurology and geriatrics at the University of Maryland. "We cannot rule out the possibility that the B vitamins may have an independent effect on the vascular cells, beyond that of lowering homocysteine," noted Dr. Macko.

While this study didn't last long enough to show a decreased risk of a second stroke, the indicators were surely there. Says Dr. Macko, "Our findings support multi-center studies which are now looking at the reduction in stroke with B vitamin therapy."

On the flip side, Tufts University investigators found that older men and women with high homocysteine and low folic acid had double the risk of narrowed carotid (neck) arteries, increasing susceptibility to strokes.

Inadequate Intakes: Americans are sadly lacking in folic acid. Thus, supplementation is the best insurance. For instance, only one in ten Americans gets the amount of folic acid experts say is needed to curb high homocysteine, according to Harvard researchers. According to Tufts research, if you get less than 350 micrograms of folic acid daily, you are apt to have high homocysteine. One study of elderly people found that those getting little folic acid (200 micrograms daily) were six times more likely to have dangerously high homocysteine than those getting more folic acid (400 micrograms daily).

What Are They and How Do They Work?

Folic Acid: Folic acid (folate), a common B vitamin, is concentrated in dried beans, orange juice, green leafy vegetables such as spinach and broccoli, cold fortified cereals, avocado, liver, and peanuts. Almost nine out of ten Americans get too little folic acid in their diets. Even so, you cannot count on high folic acid foods to curb homocysteine. In one study, a high folic acid diet did not normalize homocysteine in most subjects.

Are You At Risk for High Homocysteine?

Here's who is more apt to have high homocysteine and may need extra B vitamins:

- Low consumers of folic acid in food and supplements.
- Eaters of high-protein diets, notably animal protein, which is common in the U.S. The body makes homocysteine from protein, explains Kilmer S. McCully, M.D., at the Veterans Affairs Medical Center in Providence and originator of the homocysteine theory. Protein-rich plant foods are okay because they usually contain enough B vitamins to curb homocysteine, he adds.
- Smokers. Smoking suppresses folic acid levels, paving the way for high homocysteine. Smokers need 600 micrograms daily.
- Heavy coffee drinkers. Recent Norwegian research finds that coffee may raise homocysteine. Homocysteine was 20 percent higher in people drinking more than nine cups of coffee compared with less than one cup daily. More than five cups daily may raise homocysteine, research suggests. Those who both smoked and drank lots of coffee had particularly high homocysteine.

Of all the Bs, folic acid appears to be the most potent homocysteine fighter. Folic acid is an essential component in a process that converts homocysteine to a benign substance. Without enough folic acid, this conversion of homocysteine can't happen and levels remain high. Besides helping keep down homocysteine levels, taking folic acid while pregnant also helps prevent neural tube birth defects. Mainly for this reason, the government requires bakery products, bread, flour, pasta, and other grains to be fortified with folic acid.

Vitamin B6: Vitamin B6, also called pyridoxine, pyridoxal, and pyridoxamine, is sprinkled throughout the food supply in both plant- and animal-based foods. It's a critical player in over one hundred enzymes that affect amino acid metabolism; one of those amino acids is homocysteine.

B6 is needed to work on one of the enzymes that breaks down homocysteine. Studies consistently reveal that without enough B6 in your blood, homocysteine can build up, damaging arteries and provoking heart attacks and strokes. There's some evidence B6 also hinders dangerous blood clotting.

Vitamin B12: This vitamin is also called cobalamin, and one of its main functions is to participate in the formation of healthy red blood cells. Among other duties, B12 helps convert homocysteine to another amino acid called methionine. So you get an idea why this vitamin has been shown to help reduce blood levels of homocysteine.

Folic Acid: The Alarming Facts

- The average American over age 20 is woefully deficient in folic acid—women averaging a mere 226 micrograms of folic acid daily, men 283—far too little to curb homocysteine (or prevent cervical cancer or birth defects).
- The less folic acid in your blood, the more your arteries are apt to be narrowed and clogged, according to Tufts research.
- Smokers need three times more folic acid (at least 600 micrograms daily) to achieve the same blood levels as nonsmokers.

Folic Acid

How Much? Since it's the most important homocysteine-quasher among the B vitamins, make sure you don't skimp on this one. Dr. Malinow and other experts advise taking 400 mcg of folic acid daily to protect arteries. Smokers need 600 micrograms daily. A small percentage of people for genetic reasons need as much as 1,000 to 5,000 microgram supplements of folic acid daily to control homocysteine. Do this only with the supervision of a doctor.

Safety: Doses of 5,000 to 10,000 micrograms of folic acid daily have not caused noticeable side effects. Very high doses of folic acid could mask symptoms of B12 deficiency and pernicious anemia, unless proper diagnostic tests are used. If you have any reason to suspect you might have this condition, check it out before taking over 1,000 micrograms of folic acid a day.

Caution: If you have heart disease, consult your physician before taking high doses of B vitamins to try to correct high homocysteine.

Pills vs. Food: It's tough to get enough folic acid in food because the vitamin is poorly absorbed. A recent Irish study found that eating 400 micrograms worth of folic acid in food failed to significantly raise red blood cell levels of the vitamin. Only supplements worked. One large study found that people who did not take supplements had 10 to 15 percent higher homocysteine levels than regular multivitamin and B vitamin takers. Thus, it makes sense to eat foods rich in folic acid and to take 400 micrograms of folic acid daily—the amount common in multivitamin/mineral pills. In a recent test, heavily fortified cereals (499 to 665 micrograms of folic acid) decreased homocysteine sufficiently to prevent blood vessel damage; cereals with low folic acid (127 micrograms) did not.

Folic acid also helps prevent birth defects; mainly because of this benefit, the government recently passed a ruling requiring bakery products, bread, flour, pasta, and other grains to be fortified with folic acid. Since then, researchers have detected higher levels of folic acid in the blood of Americans.

Vitamin B6

How Much? Typical multivitamin pills contain 3 milligrams of B6, which is enough to correct deficiencies and boost immunity. Supplements of 10 to 50 milligrams of B6 a day may be more effective to reduce homocysteine, studies show.

Safety: It's safest to stick to a dose of no more than 50 milligrams of B6 daily. Avoid doses of more than 200 milligrams a day. High doses, especially over the long term, can cause neurological symptoms. Doses of 500 to 1,000 milligrams daily have produced nervous system toxicity.

Pills vs. Food: While it's important to eat foods rich in B6, it is difficult to get the homocysteine-preventing doses from diet alone. In fact, the average B6 intake in this country is 1.79 milligrams, according to a recent U.S. Department of Agriculture survey.

Vitamin B12

How Much? In Dr. David Spence's study showing the homocysteine-lowering effects of B vitamins, people were given 250 micrograms of B12. Because many people as they age lose the ability to absorb B12 from food, some experts recommend fairly high doses to overcome this problem. From 250 to 500 micrograms daily should offer heart protection.

Safety: B12 appears to be very safe. Research studies have used 1,000 to 5,000 micrograms daily without seeing side effects. Although toxicity is very low, don't exceed 1,000 micrograms daily except on the advice of a doctor.

Pills vs. Foods: While vegetarians generally have a leg up on the rest of the population in terms of diet, the one nutrient that they could be low in is vitamin B12, since it is found only in foods of animal origin. Fortunately, most fortified cereals include B12, making things easier for strict vegans. However, vegetarian or not, it would be difficult to get the levels used in the homocysteine research without taking a supplement.

Chapter 4

Calcium: Beyond Bones

Why play Russian roulette with your blood pressure when calcium can do so much?

Our Stone Age ancestors ate lots of calcium. And you don't. They ate 2,000 to 3,000 milligrams a day of calcium, mostly from foraged wild plants. That's five times more than today's average of about 600 milligrams for women ages 35 to 75, according to a large-scale government survey. Our bodies were designed by evolution to run on extraordinarily high amounts of calcium compared with the paltry amounts we get today. Moreover, the deficiency worsens with age, as we tend to absorb less calcium with the passing years.

We all know calcium is essential for developing and maintaining strong bones. But what's less well known is its essential role in maintaining a healthy heart.

What Is It?

Calcium is the most abundant mineral in the body; we need at least 1,000 milligrams of it daily compared to a few milligrams or even micrograms of most other vitamins and minerals. Calcium makes up about 2 percent of body weight; 99 percent is in bones, teeth, and other hard tissue. But that 1 percent floating in the blood and fluids means a lot to your heart.

The Evidence

Blood Pressure: Calcium may save you from high blood pressure as you get older, and is particularly effective in older people, notably those who are salt sensitive. Blood pressure rises in response to eating too much sodium. In a recent review of all studies in which subjects with high blood pressure took calcium supplements, David A. McCarron, M.D., Oregon Health Sciences University, noted that the calcium tablets depressed blood pressure in 75 percent of the cases. It dropped an average 5 to 7 mm/Hg for systolic (upper number) and 3 to 4 mm/Hg for diastolic. The doses ranged from 400 milligrams to 2,000 milligrams daily and usually were taken for six to twelve weeks.

A high calcium intake may prevent the onset of high blood pressure in the first place. Investigators at Boston University Medical School recently tracked a large group of men for eighteen years. Those who ate the most calcium (up to 1,100 milligrams a day) were 20 percent less apt to develop high blood pressure as they aged than those eating the least (under 110 milligrams a day). Another study of nonoverweight, moderate drinkers under age 40 showed that taking in 1,000 milligrams of calcium daily cut their risk of developing high blood pressure in later years by 40 percent.

If everyone took calcium supplements, blood pressure would drop in about 50 percent of Americans, says hypertension researcher Lawrence M. Resnick, M.D., of Wayne State University in Detroit.

More remarkable, calcium may reverse some of high blood pressure's damage. Years of elevated blood pressure can result in strokes, left ventricular hypertrophy (enlargement of the left chamber of the heart), and congestive heart failure. Wayne State investigators found that taking a daily 1,000 milligrams of calcium carbonate for eight weeks caused enlarged hearts to diminish in size!

Cholesterol Buster: Surprisingly, calcium may be a weapon against bad cholesterol. In a test by Margo A. Denke, of the University of Texas Southwestern Medical Center in Dallas, men with moderately high cholesterol ate a diet fairly high in beef and fat and low in calcium—410 milligrams daily. Then they switched to a high-calcium regimen of 2,200 milligrams per day. Their average total cholesterol dipped 6 percent. More important, their artery-clogging bad LDL cholesterol fell 11 percent.

How Does It Work?

Its most famous role is setting the framework for bone, but it's the tiny percent of calcium in blood and fluids that affects the heart. Calcium works with enzymes responsible for muscle contraction and nerve transmission, helping regulate heartbeat. Calcium affects blood pressure in different ways: it is essential for the proper workings of the muscle cells and hormones that cause blood vessels to contract.

Calcium fights cholesterol by partially deterring the absorption of cholesterol-raising saturated fat from our intestinal tracts. The less saturated fat you absorb from cheese, cream, fatty meats, and other foods high in saturated fat, the less cholesterol you'll make. In one study, twice as much fat washed out in the men's stools during the high-calcium diets. Don't rely on calcium to protect you from a high-fat diet, but it may lessen the blow.

How Much? To prevent or correct high blood pressure or high cholesterol, you may need high doses of up to 2,000 milligrams of calcium per day. Since these are therapeutic doses, consult your doctor before taking such high doses, especially if you are taking medications.

Safety: Too much calcium can trigger either of two opposite ends of intestinal discomfort: constipation or diarrhea. To prevent either problem, drink lots of water, and space pills throughout the day. Don't take more than 500 to 600 milligrams at one time for best absorption. The latest National Academy of Sciences recommendation advises limiting calcium to no more than 2,500 mg daily.

Contrary to popular belief, neither calcium nor vitamin C promotes formation of kidney stones, recent studies find. Actually, there's evidence that supplements of either may help retard growth of the stones.

Pills vs. Food: Unless you religiously eat several

servings a day of high-calcium foods, such as dairy products, canned sardines or salmon, leafy green vegetables, tofu, or calcium-fortified foods, you need a supplement. But then again, why take chances? Calcium supplements are cheap, effective, and reliable, says Harvard's Walter Willett. Usually a separate tablet is needed because multivitamin/mineral pills rarely contain enough calcium. Even if you are on hypertension medication, calcium supplements can induce further drops in blood pressure, says Dr. McCarron. But, he cautions, be sure to inform your physician if you start taking calcium supplements on top of medication.

What Kind? Don't take calcium supplements made of bonemeal or dolomite. They can contain dangerous amounts of lead. Best choices: calcium carbonate and calcium citrate. Be sure to check the label for the amount of pure or elemental calcium each tablet delivers. This tells the amount of usable calcium in the pill, and is the only way to know how much calcium you are really getting from a specific pill. Supplements differ greatly. For example, calcium gluconate contains only 9 percent elemental calcium; calcium carbonate has 40 percent. Tums are pure calcium carbonate, thus identical to a calcium supplement. Research at Tufts shows that a newer form of calcium called calcium citrate malate is exceptionally potent, about 40 percent more absorbable. Thus, you need much less to match the impact of other calcium supplements.

Chapter 5

Magnificent Magnesium

Chances are great that you don't get enough magnesium to protect cells against premature heart aging. Thus, your heart is apt to give out at an earlier age, you are more apt to have a heart attack, and you're more apt to be plagued by chronic high blood pressure.

Don't risk premature heart disease and cutting your life short just because you don't get enough magnesium. It's a youth-preserving mineral, especially for your heart. Even small shortages of magnesium appear to make a difference in heart health and general aging. For one thing, as you age you tend to eat diets lower in magnesium, and worse, absorb less of it. That lack can accelerate the heart disease and aging process, as animal studies strikingly illustrate. Animals made deficient in magnesium age more rapidly and die earlier. Depriving young animals of magnesium creates vascular changes and neuromuscular abnormalities typical in aged animals. Indeed, magnesium-starved animals are nearly perfect specimens of accelerated aging, say French researchers. Giving animals magnesium supplements prevents these changes.

If you chronically have suboptimal levels of magnesium, you too can expect to show the risk factors for heart disease earlier: in particular, clogged arteries, heart arrhythmias (irregular heartbeats), heart attacks, high blood pressure, and insulin resistance possibly leading to diabetes.

What Is It?

We carry about an ounce of magnesium in our bodies; most of it's in bone and muscles, about 15 percent stays in blood and other fluids. It's sprinkled throughout both plant and animal foods; dark greens are a great source, since magnesium is an essential part of chlorophyll. So are cereal grains and legumes.

The Alarming Facts

- On average, Americans get only three-fourths the recommended dietary allowance for magnesium, even though the RDA is far too low to begin with, say many experts.
- Older people, who need it most, get less. Older men barely get two-thirds of the RDA, older women just 70 percent.
- You're not likely to get enough magnesium from food unless you eat at least 2,000 calories a day.

The Evidence

Evidence pours in that too little magnesium makes you more susceptible to heart disease. Over the long haul, magnesium deficiency causes all sorts of heart problems, such as arrhythmias and high blood pressure.

Fends Off Heart Disease: A recent study of 15,000 men and women, ages 45 to 64, by University of Minnesota researchers found that those with existing cardiovascular disease, high blood pressure, and diabetes had significantly lower blood levels of magnesium than those free of such diseases. Women with low blood levels of magnesium were more apt to have high bad type LDL cholesterol and thickening of the walls of carotid (neck) arteries, indicating clogged arteries. Those with high dietary and blood magnesium had higher good type HDL cholesterol as well as lower levels of blood sugar and insulin, a hormone that damages artery walls.

People who take in low amounts of magnesium are more apt to have heart disease, according to "about twenty worldwide population studies," says Ronald J. Elin, M.D., a magnesium authority at the National Institutes of Health. Magnesium seems to protect the heart several different ways, in particular by preventing spasms of the coronary arteries and abnormal heart rhythms that are a primary cause of sudden death. In one study of a cardiac unit, 53 percent of the patients had low magnesium. Indeed, the amount of magnesium in your body can help determine whether you live or die if you have a heart attack.

Discourages Clots: Further, magnesium helps deter formation of blood clots that help clog arteries and trigger heart attacks. Specifically, studies by Jerry L. Nadler, M.D., at City of Hope Medical Center in Duarte, California, show that magnesium inhibits release of thromboxane, a substance that makes blood platelets more sticky and apt to form clots. The mineral also tends to keep blood vessels from constricting, thus warding off rises in blood pressure, strokes, and heart attacks. Magnesium has been so effective in regulating heartbeat and blood pressure that it has been called "nature's calcium channel blocker," referring to prescription calcium blocker drugs used for those purposes.

Lowers Blood Pressure: In experiments where people are temporarily deprived of magnesium in the diet, blood pressure rises. And a major Harvard study found that those getting low amounts of magnesium were more apt to develop high blood pressure. A recent Swedish study found a dramatic drop in blood pressure from taking magnesium supplements. After nine weeks, systolic (upper number) blood pressure went down from 154 to 146 and diastolic (lower number) pressure from 100 to 92 in patients taking about 360 milligrams of magnesium daily. In another study by Dutch researchers at Erasmus University Medical School in Rotterdam, middle-aged and elderly women with mild to moderate high blood pressure took magnesium supplements (485 milligrams a day) for six months. Their systolic blood pressure fell 2.7 mm/Hg and diastolic blood pressure fell 3.4 mm/Hg lower than that of women taking a dummy pill.

Curbs Free Radicals: Recent investigations by a team of scientists at the Center for Research on Human Nutrition at France's National Institute of Agricultural Research suggest that the root cause of heart disease and rapid aging induced by a magnesium deficiency is increased free radical activity in cells. They find cells from magnesium-deficient animals more prone to free radical damage. Such cells' membranes become rigid, destroying cell integrity and disrupting the proper flow of calcium through membranes. This "uncontrolled calcium inflow," suspect French researchers, is a "central event in the aging process and cell injury."

Animals low in magnesium also release greater amounts of highly inflammatory agents called cytokines that in turn create more free radicals and subsequent cell damage and inflammation in the arteries. Long-term magnesium deficiency also robs the body of one of its principal heart protectors—vitamin E—probably because so much is used up trying to fend off increased free radical attacks.

Worst of all, the mitochondria, the energy factories of the cells particularly critical in heart function, are increasingly damaged in the absence of adequate magnesium. When you mess with mitochondria, you disrupt the very crux of a cell's life, the ability to create energy. Thus, the heart grows weaker.

Prevents and Reverses Diabetes: Since the high levels of blood sugar and insulin in diabetes damages arteries, anything that helps ward off this condition also helps the heart. Evidence is popping up linking diabetes with a deficiency of magnesium. Further, fairly low doses of magnesium may help prevent diabetic complications and intervene in the course of the disease itself. The theory is that diabetics have a peculiar defect in the metabolism of magnesium. Studies find that most diabetics often have low levels of magnesium in their cells and blood. This is worrisome, because a lack of magnesium can encourage blood clotting, constriction of blood vessels, high blood pressure, irregular heartbeats, and insulin resistance, according to Robert K. Rude, M.D., associate professor of medicine at the University of Southern California. He favors 300 to 400 milligram supplements daily, preferably of magnesium chloride, to correct diabetic deficiencies. Diabetes, he says, is characterized by magnesium depletion.

Postscript: Even if you don't have diabetes or heart disease, skimping on magnesium can make you more vulnerable to insulin resistance—a condition you don't want. In one study of normal healthy individuals, all developed a 25 percent greater insulin resistance on a magnesium-deficient diet. Such a sluggish abnormal functioning of insulin can eventually damage arteries and possibly bring on diabetes.

Stretches Life: You're more apt to survive a heart attack if you don't skimp on magnesium. A recent ten-year study of 2,182 men in Wales found that those eating magnesium-low diets had one and a half times the risk of sudden death from heart attacks as those eating one-third more magnesium. Also, the high magnesium eaters were only half as likely to have any type of cardiovascular incident such as nonfatal heart attack, stroke, angina (chest pain), or heart surgery. The protective average difference in magnesium intake was only an extra 30 milligrams—the amount in half an ounce of almonds.

The Heart-Protective Promise of Magnesium

- Reduces vascular spasms
- Reduces angina (chest pain)
- Increases clot-busting activity
- Inhibits blood platelet stickiness leading to clots
- Helps keep heartbeats normal
- Boosts good types of blood cholesterol (HDLs and APO A1)
- Suppresses triglycerides

How Does It Work?

This mineral really gets around; magnesium is a necessary part of over three hundred enzyme systems in the body. Among other things, magnesium is involved in muscle contraction (including heart muscle), nervous system transmission, and the body's protein and DNA production. There are so many ways that magnesium can affect the heart: it's necessary for heartbeat, it works on the contraction and relaxation of blood vessels, it can help reduce plaque buildup in arteries, and it also helps prevent blood clots.

What to Take

How Much? Your total daily accumulation should be 500 milligrams; a balanced diet should give you at least 200 to 300 mg (more if it's very rich in greens and bran), so a separate supplement of 200 to 300 milligrams should be enough. A typical multivitamin/ mineral pill contains about 100 milligrams. So if you opt for more, you need a separate magnesium tablet.

Safety: More than 600 to 700 milligrams daily of elemental magnesium can cause diarrhea. Magnesium experts consider a daily dose of 500 milligrams of elemental magnesium per day extremely safe for the average individual with normal kidney function. (However, the National Academy of Sciences recommends no more than 350 mg of magnesium per day from supplements, and sets no upper limit for magnesium from food.)

Warning: Don't take magnesium supplements if you have kidney problems or severe heart failure. And stop taking supplements if you develop diarrhea. If you have already had a heart attack, consult your physician before taking magnesium.

Pills vs. Food: Actually, you can get lots of magnesium if you eat whole grains, dark greens, nuts, seeds, and legumes. However, supplementing is probably necessary, especially if you don't eat magnesium-rich foods.

What Type? Magnesium chloride, magnesium aspartate, magnesium gluconate, and magnesium lactate all seem to be absorbed well and are better tolerated by most people than magnesium oxide. A type called Slo-mag is preferred by many experts.

Chapter 6

Selenium: Heart Protector

While protecting your heart, this powerhouse antioxidant safeguards the rest of your body from the ravages of aging.

Selenium's diverse antiaging properties includes protection from heart disease. When your cells get low in selenium—as they tend to do with age—your immune functioning goes awry and you are more apt to fall prey to heart disease, infections, and cancer. Further, selenium is not only an antioxidant on its own, it is an essential building block for the creation of glutathione peroxidase, one of the body's most critical enzymes. Some researchers believe much of selenium's antiaging power is due to its ability to boost production of this free radical–fighting enzyme.

What Is It?

Unlike calcium and magnesium, which your body stores in fairly large amounts, selenium is a trace mineral, present in minute amounts in your tissues. Instead of a gram or milligram requirement, we need only microgram amounts of selenium in the diet

(1 microgram is a millionth of a gram). Still, this mineral is absolutely essential to growth and health, and a giant in the area of disease prevention.

How Does It Work?

The activity of one of the body's important free radical fighters—the enzyme glutathione peroxidase—is dependent on selenium. Glutathione peroxidase destroys free radicals that trigger the formation of plaque that clogs arteries leading to the heart.

The Evidence

Lowers Heart Disease Risk: Low blood levels of selenium make you more vulnerable to heart disease, studies show. A large-scale Finnish study found that those with the lowest blood levels of selenium were three times more apt to die of heart disease than those with the highest blood levels of selenium.

Another study found that the lower your blood selenium, the greater the degree of blockage in arteries as determined by angiograms (heart X rays). Apparently, selenium can save your heart in several ways. It protects arteries by preventing platelet aggregation that tends to form blood clots, triggering heart attacks and strokes. Selenium also helps block oxidation of bad type LDL cholesterol, thought to be the primary step in artery clogging.

Selenium also protects your heart from viral infections. A lack of selenium may allow viruses to run rampant in your body, according to recent research at the U.S. Department of Agriculture. In mice raised on diets deficient in selenium (or vitamin E), a normally harmless virus mutated into a virulent one, inflicting serious damage on heart muscle. "It was a viral transformation from Dr. Jekyll to Mr. Hyde," says USDA's Orville A. Levander.

The Alarming Facts

- As you age, your levels of selenium fall. Selenium blood levels dropped 7 percent after age 60, and 24 percent after age 75, according to Italian research.
- Declining selenium signifies less antioxidant activity in your blood and tissues.
- People with low levels of selenium have more heart disease, cancer, and arthritis.

How Much? For protection, you need from 100 to 200 micrograms a day, says Dr. Donald J. Lisk at Cornell University. He has also sampled the potency of many selenium supplements on the market and found them to be excellent. You don't have to worry that they deliver more than or less than the label claims, he says.

Safety: Selenium can be toxic (hair loss, liver damage, joint inflammation) in high doses, so don't overdose on supplements. Even excessively eating Brazil nuts could be toxic to the liver, as animal experiments have shown. But to get a toxic effect, you would have to eat as much as 2,500 micrograms of selenium a day, says Dr. Lisk. Japanese fishermen get over 500 micrograms a day without apparent harm. Inhabitants in China have developed severe toxic symptoms after 5,000 micrograms of selenium a day. There is no reason to go above 200 micrograms per day, which experts say is safe.

Pills vs. Food: You get selenium in grains, sunflower seeds, meat, seafood—especially tuna, swordfish, and oysters—and garlic. But for a major injection of selenium, nothing beats Brazil nuts, grown in the selenium-rich soil of the forests of the Amazon. Unless you're eating lots of Brazil nuts, you need to supplement.

Chapter 7

Iron: Heart Enemy

Here's one mineral that can actually damage your heart. Too much iron can contribute to heart disease and aging by fostering free radical attacks on cells. Don't routinely take iron supplements if you are an adult male or a woman past menopause.

Iron-poor blood. Tired blood. Iron-deficiency anemia. Such are the feared consequences of too little iron. But a greater danger for most men and older women is too much iron. Taking iron supplements and stuffing yourself with iron-rich foods can wreck your mission to prevent or reverse heart disease. High tissue stores of iron, especially past middle age, are more apt to make you sick and old than to keep you young and vital.

"Excess iron can be very dangerous," explains prominent researcher on aging Dr. Denham Harman of the University of Nebraska, because it facilitates free radical damage to cells. For example, iron helps change benign LDL cholesterol into the toxic type that wrecks arteries and makes hearts fail. Iron also aggravates the intensity of free radical reactions, furthering fierce free radical chain reactions that rip through many cells.

Startling evidence from a 1992 Finnish study showed that men with the most iron in their blood were twice as likely to have heart attacks as men with the least iron-rich blood. (Iron was extra-hazardous to men with high blood cholesterol.) A later Harvard study zeroed in on heme iron, found in meat and better absorbed than vegetable iron, as a culprit. Men with the most blood heme iron had 50 percent higher odds of heart attack than men with the least heme iron. Although the idea that iron might foster heart disease struck some as wacky, antiaging researchers were not surprised. Some had been preaching for more than a decade that iron is in cahoots with free radicals to do you in.

Although some studies have not identified iron as a culprit in heart disease, the role of iron and other metals in fostering free radical reactions provides compelling theoretical reasons to incriminate the metal in cell damage, aging, and chronic diseases, including heart disease.

It makes sense that iron can be toxic, insists Jerome Sullivan, a pathologist at the Veteran Affairs Medical Center in Charleston, South Carolina, who first proposed the theory in 1981. He argues that the risk of heart attack rises in direct proportion to the amount of iron stored in the body. For example, he points out that men start having heart attacks in their 20s, after they are fully grown and begin to pile up iron in the blood and liver. In contrast, premenopausal women who lose iron every month through menstruation are oddly protected from heart attacks. They succumb after menopause, when menstruation stops and iron builds up in the blood—although, of course, other factors such as estrogen may be involved.

According to Dr. Sullivan, there is no physiological reason whatever to encourage women after menopause or grown men to try to raise their bodily stores of iron. All you need is an adequate low-maintenance dose to keep things running smoothly, he says.

Five Ways to Avoid Excess Iron if You Are a Woman Past Menopause or a Man

1. Don't take individual iron supplements. Look for multivitamin/mineral tablets with low amounts of iron or no iron—certainly no more than 100 percent of the RDA. Beware that some multi formulas have alarmingly high amounts of iron—as much as 40 milligrams, more than 200 percent of the RDA.
2. Cut down on animal foods. You absorb the heme iron in meat much more readily than the nonheme iron in vegetables such as beans and cereals. Red meat is particularly bad, says Emory University researcher Dr. Dean Jones, because it combines high iron with high fat—a perfect setting for the production of peroxides and free radicals. Indeed, a Harvard study by Dr. Alberto Ascherio found that men eating the most heme or red meat iron had a 43 percent higher risk of heart attack than those

eating the least heme iron. It's riskier to get your iron from meat than from cereal, he says.

3. Consume foods and beverages that tend to block absorption of iron, such as tea, red wine, and high-fiber bran and beans. This could be yet another reason tea drinkers tend to live longer, red wine drinkers seem to have less heart disease, and fiber helps frustrate cancer. All three contain chemicals that limit iron's ability to foster cell-damaging interactions with free radicals.

4. Beware of iron-fortified cereals. Some cereals such as Total and Product 19 contain 18 milligrams of iron per serving—100 percent of the Daily Value, the level used by the food labels, which is the highest RDA for any age/sex group. Note: Such cereals are okay, indeed beneficial, for younger women and children, who are often low in iron.

5. If you are a man of any age or a woman past menopause, you might also help protect yourself by donating blood three times a year to deplete unwanted iron stores.

Caution: Menstruating women tend to lose iron regularly in blood flow and may need iron supplements. Also, children and adolescents often do not get enough iron, and may need iron supplements.

Chapter 8

Coenzyme Q-10: Amazing Heart Energizer

It's a heart medicine used around the world, and if your doctor doesn't know about it, you can easily get it on your own; it could save your life.

If you have heart problems, you should know about a substance called coenzyme Q-10. It appears to be a powerful reenergizer of heart cells and can bring new hope to millions of people with heart disease, particularly those with congestive heart failure, in which heart muscle steadily weakens, causing the heart's pumping function to deteriorate. The condition is very common, especially in older people, and may not respond to conventional treatments. It stems from various causes: long-standing high blood pressure, diabetes, viral diseases, alcohol abuse, and most frequently, a heart attack or just plain everyday damage from the aging process. Impaired, the tiny heart cells no longer generate enough energy to orchestrate the forceful heart contractions that pump blood throughout the body. Because of heart muscle cells' inefficiency, blood flow slows and heart function begins to fail. "Literally, heart failure is an energy-starved heart," says one cardiologist. Typical symptoms are shortness of breath, fatigue, fluid in the lungs, and swelling of the ankles. Gradually, the overworked heart may give out and shut down, leading to the body's steady deterioration and death. Congestive heart failure is epidemic in Western countries. It's the number one reason for hospitalization in older Americans. Common treatment: drugs such as digitalis, diuretics, vasodilators, and ACE inhibitors. The ultimate cure: heart transplant. But there's another common treatment that's used throughout the world with great success. It reenergizes the heart by giving cells a renewed burst of energy. It's called coenzyme Q-10, and its miracles are legendary among some cardiologists.

What Is It?

Coenzyme Q-10 is a strong antioxidant known also as ubiquinol-10. It has been described as "vitaminlike," but some experts say it is definitely a vitamin—that is, a nutrient your body must take in to feed your cells so your body can operate at an optimum level. It is present in very small amounts in food, notably seafood, and is produced by all cells of the body. Japanese scientists have synthesized coQ-10 into a raw material that is put into supplements and sold throughout the world by several Japanese companies.

The Evidence

Compelling evidence shows that most heart patients are deficient in coQ-10 and that taking coQ-10 supplements revitalizes heart function and can dramatically relieve heart disease symptoms. Pioneering studies by the late Karl Folkers, Ph.D., then director of the Institute for Biomedical Research at the University of Texas at Austin, showed that 75 percent of heart patients have severe deficiencies of coQ-10 in heart tissue compared with healthy individuals. Further, he documented that taking coenzyme Q-10 significantly benefited three-fourths of a group of elderly patients with congestive heart failure. More than fifty major articles have been published in reputable medical journals worldwide in the last ten years on the use of coQ-10 for heart disease, primarily congestive heart failure.

Extensive Japanese research has found that about 70 percent of patients improved on coQ-10. CoQ-10 is also widely used in Italy, having been tested in trials at several centers involving 2,500 patients. Eighty percent of heart-failure patients improved after taking 100 milligrams of coQ-10 along with conventional therapy. In a follow-up study, 50 milligrams of coQ-10 daily for a month, alone or with other treatments, significantly improved symptoms of heart failure and quality of life. Because of the international research on coQ-10, it is a drug of choice in many countries. It is "routinely" given to patients with congestive heart failure in Israeli hospitals. Japanese doctors have used coQ-10 for cardiac problems for more than thirty years. It is now among the top six pharmaceutical agents used in Japan. If you have heart failure in Italy, it's likely to be recommended.

Dr. Stephen T. Sinatra, an assistant clinical professor at the University of Connecticut School of Medicine, is one of a growing number of American physicians using coQ-10. "I personally use Q-10 for every one of my patients with congestive heart failure if they are willing to take it," he says. He has treated thousands of heart patients with coQ-10, and he estimates it has helped more than 70 percent of them. Some of his failures, he believes, were due to doses that were inadequate or products without sufficient potency. The dose must be enough to substantially raise blood levels of coQ-10; if that happens, he believes, about 100 percent of heart patients would benefit.

In one case of an elderly woman with congestive heart failure, Dr. Sinatra saw no improvement from a typically prescribed daily dose of 90 milligrams of coQ-10. However, increasing the daily dose to 300 milligrams produced remarkable improvement in heart functioning. Dr. Sinatra now recommends trying higher doses if lower ones do not work.

Lowers Blood Pressure: Taking an average 225 milligrams of coQ-10 daily reduced blood pressure in about 85 percent of 109 patients with high blood pressure, according to a recent study by Texas cardiologist Peter Langsjoen, M.D., in cooperation with researchers at the University of Texas at Austin.

CoQ-10 caused no blood pressure changes in 15 percent of patients, and one patient got worse. Generally, however, taking coQ-10 pushed systolic (upper number) pressure down from 159 to 147, and diastolic pressure from 94 to 85, usually within three or four months. Further, echocardiograms (heart ultrasound pictures) found improvements in heart function. Most important, at the start of the study nearly all patients were on antihypertensive drugs. After coQ-10 treatment, 51 percent of the patients were able to completely stop taking from one to three of their antihypertensive medications and 25 percent were able to control their blood pressure with coQ-10 alone.

Saves Arteries: Coenzyme Q-10 strikes at the root cause of atherosclerosis. It is exceptionally strong in halting the relentless oxidation of blood cholesterol that is the first step in making a rotten mess of your arteries, precipitating heart attacks and strokes. According to Boston University researcher Balz Frei, ubiquinol-10 prevents artery-destroying oxidation of LDL bad type cholesterol much more efficiently than either vitamin E, which is an acknowledged antioxidant heavyweight in this arena, or beta carotene. However, coQ-10 is quickly consumed during this process, so having lots on hand is critical in keeping arteries unclogged and young. Since fatty fish is the best dietary source of coQ-10, this may help explain why fish eaters have healthier arteries.

Mainstream medicine is becoming more interested in the heart-saving potential of coQ-10, namely because of patient reports and the accumulating scientific evidence that it works. Dr. Michael Sole, a professor of medicine at the University of Toronto and director of the Per Munk Cardiac Centre, one of the world's largest and most prominent centers for the treatment and study of heart disease, says it's time to seriously investigate coQ-10. He has begun studies to try to determine exactly what it does in the heart.

Dr. Sole confesses that his interest was piqued by an experience with a patient who needed a pacemaker, didn't get one, but recovered anyway. "I had this patient with a deteriorating heart condition who developed a heart block and needed a pacemaker," says Dr. Sole. "I referred him to get one implanted, but when I saw him four months later, he hadn't had his pacemaker put in. To my surprise, his condition, which had been deteriorating over the last several years, had remarkably reversed itself. So I said to him, 'Wow, this is amazing! I've never seen anything like this in my entire experience as a cardiologist.' At which point the patient confessed to me he didn't want a pacemaker and after seeing me had talked to a friend who was taking coenzyme Q-10, so he decided to take it himself." Was the coQ-10 responsible or coincidental in this startling case? As Dr. Sole says, it is merely one case, and he doesn't know the answer. "But it was dramatic enough to make me wonder. Of course, I've seen miracles come and go, and whether coQ-10 is one is something we need to explore by doing the type of double-blind controlled studies that will tell us for sure. At the moment, it sure looks promising enough to be worthy of our further investigation."

How Does It Work?

CoQ-10 is a unique antioxidant that reportedly penetrates the cells' tiny "energy factories," called mitochondria, where oxygen is burned, giving cells energy to carry on the business of life. To efficiently burn energy, the mitochondria need coQ-10. It is often called the "spark" that starts and helps drive the mitochondrial engines.

Without enough coQ-10, the theory goes, cells suffer power shortages, impairing the function of vital organs, most noticeably the heart, which needs the most coQ-10 to generate the tremendous energy needed to keep the heart beating. When damaged heart muscle cells are depleted of vital coQ-10, energy production is low, resulting in mitochondrial and cardiovascular dysfunction. Supplying the heart muscle with coQ-10 supplements revitalizes energy-starved cells, boosting power output, leading to a more efficient heart that doesn't have to work so hard to circulate blood, say experts. In short, coQ-10 improves mechanical function of the heart by giving energy-starved cells the fuel needed to function efficiently. CoQ-10 may also help prevent and heal degenerative damage to heart cells and help keep bad LDL cholesterol from clogging arteries.

How Much? A typical dose for heart disease is 50 to 150 milligrams a day; however, up to 300 milligrams a day may be needed when heart failure is severe. Dr. Sinatra says that the sicker the cardiac patient, the weaker the heart, the higher the coQ-10 dose needs to be. Some researchers recommend 2 milligrams of coQ-10 for each kilogram (2.2 pounds) of body weight. Critically important is the fact that, to be effective, the dose of coQ-10 must significantly raise blood levels of coQ-10. The amount needed to do that varies among individuals, and also depends on the potency or bioavailability of the coQ-10 used. Some people get a good rise with 100 milligrams, whereas others need two or three times that much to attain the same blood level, says internationally known cardiologist-researcher Peter H. Langsjoen in Bullard, Texas, who uses coQ-10 extensively in his practice and has done research with Dr. Folkers.

The only way to be sure if coQ-10 is working, and to determine what dose is needed, is to measure blood levels, he says.

How Quickly Does It Work? Typically, it takes two to eight weeks for coQ-10 to produce an improvement in symptoms of heart failure, say authorities. You must take coQ-10 continually to maintain its heart-strengthening benefits. It is not a permanent, short-time cure.

Safety: Side effects are minor and rare, usually nothing more than mild transient nausea. In the large Italian study, 22 out of 2,664 patients reported mild side effects, or slightly less than 1 percent. No toxicity has been found, even at high doses, in animals or humans, says Dr. Folkers.

Caution: Remember that coQ-10 is not a substitute for conventional drugs, but is usually used along with conventional therapy for best results. CoQ-10 may allow you to reduce dosage of conventional drugs, but you should do this with the supervision of your doctor. Although many people with varying degrees of atherosclerosis, which virtually all adults have by middle age, may want to take coQ-10 as a preventive, heart failure is a serious condition that should not be self-diagnosed or self-medicated. If you have serious heart disease, always consult a doctor for the proper course of treatment.

How to Take: All coQ-10 is made in Japan and sold to numerous companies that package it in pressed tablets, powder-filled capsules, or gel caps. Because coQ-10 is fat-soluble, it's essential to take dry coQ-10 with some fat for absorption. If you simply gulp down a dry coQ-10 tablet, much of it is wasted. One cardiologist suggests taking it with a little peanut butter or olive oil. Some companies now produce coQ-10 in soft gel capsules, claiming it is better absorbed. You can also get chewable coQ-10 pills that have far higher bioavailability than plain dry powdered tablets you swallow, says Dr. Langsjoen. A chewable wafer he uses personally and has been used in research studies is available from the Vitaline Corp. in Ashland, Oregon, (800-648-4755). Unfortunately, coQ-10, partly because of the Japanese monopoly, is relatively costly.

Chapter 9

OPC: Blood Vessel Fixer

It may cure many ills, but there's nothing like it for strengthening blood vessels and fighting varicose veins.

It's your lifeline—that intricate network of blood vessels, from tiny capillaries to large arteries and veins, that feeds blood to every bit of tissue from the top of your head to the tip of your toes. The integrity and strength of these blood vessels, combined with the proper functioning of your heart, are unquestionably paramount factors in your health and survival. If blood vessels grow old or diseased, fragile, thin, and leaky, your heart—as well as your overall health—is compromised. If blood-carrying oxygen doesn't flow through properly, your heart muscle can be damaged, your brain cells may die or malfunction, your leg muscles may cramp and cause pain, your vision may diminish. If a blood vessel leaks or bursts, you may suffer a brain hemorrhage or "bleeding stroke," or tiny spider veins may appear on the surface of your skin. Your gums and nose may bleed; varicose veins may bulge in your legs. Fluid may leak through permeable blood vessels, causing swelling or edema. Nothing is more critical than the vitality of those miles of capillaries, veins, and arteries that make up your circulatory system.

Yet, has anyone ever told you of a medicine that can actually strengthen fragile and weakened blood vessels, restoring them to normal health, reversing and preventing circulatory disasters?

There is such a unique natural remedy—a drug extensively used in Europe with amazing success. There's no other medicine like it anywhere. And you can easily get it.

OPC, as it's commonly called in scientific circles, is expert at treating vascular diseases because it actually increases the structural strength of weakened blood vessels. It also has other biological activity and is one of the most potent antioxidants known—fifty times as powerful as vitamin E, according to some tests. Antioxidants can help neutralize the underlying chemical cause (free radicals) that promotes most diseases.

Research on OPC is just beginning in the United States, so there are few scientific data in American medical journals or textbooks to back up therapeutic claims. But there are four decades of proven use in Europe, especially France, to be excited about. Many Americans are already raving about the wondrous relief they have experienced from taking OPC, and its popularity is sure to soar as its benefits become even better known. Some experts call OPC a superstar among botanical supplements, the one with the most potential of all for benefiting human health.

What Is It?

Derived commercially from grape seeds and the bark of the pine tree, it is a mixture of antioxidant molecules, variously called proanthocyanidins, pro-cyanidins, proanthocyanidolic oligomers (PCO), oligomeric procyanidins (OPC), pycnogenols (generic), Pycnogenol™ (pronounced pik-NOD-ja-nol), or just plain grape seed extract.

In 1947 the renowned French chemist Jack Masquelier, professor emeritus of medicine at the University of Bordeaux, isolated the first OPC, a colorless substance, from the red skin of the peanut. He tells how he gave it to the wife of the dean of his faculty, who had severe edema from pregnancy; her legs had gotten so swollen, she could barely walk. "Well, the dean's wife was cured in forty-eight hours," says Dr. Masquelier. "So there had to be something special about my extract." In 1950 the peanut-skin OPC became the first vasculo-protective medicine, known as Resivit and sold in France. About a quarter of a century later another drug based on Dr. Masquelier's grape seed OPC, called Endotelon, made its debut in France. By 1979 Masquelier had also christened his brainchild "pycnogenols," a generic word describing in Greek its multifaceted chemistry. (Later the term "Pycnogenol" became a patented registered trademark of a British company, Horphag Research Limited.) Dr. Masquelier also has detected OPC in virtually all plants, red wine, and the peanut kernel itself. The current concentrated commercial sources are grape seeds and the bark of the French maritime pine tree. Dr. Masquelier also says OPC primarily accounts for the antioxidant, artery-protecting activity of red wine and tea.

The Evidence

If you lived in France, you might know OPC best as a foremost drug to treat varicose veins, a potentially disfiguring, painful condition in which veins tend to sag and stretch, become inflamed, and appear as purplish, elongated bulges beneath the skin. Taking OPC, studies show, can actually strengthen the veins, firming them up and restoring their resilience so they retract back into the skin. Dr. Masquelier and colleagues have done nine studies confirming OPC's efficacy for varicose veins. Another primary use of OPC is to reduce fluid buildup, or edema. When vascular walls become weakened, fluids transported inside the veins leak out, leading to swelling. By strengthening capillary walls and performing other biological maneuvers, OPC reduces edema and swelling, which may be important in fighting high blood pressure, congestive heart failure, and sports injuries involving swelling. Additionally, OPC has been used to treat eye problems—glare, night blindness, macular degeneration—arthritis, hay fever and allergies, and nosebleeds.

"If you regularly take OPC, your vascular walls will be reinforced," says Dr. Masquelier. He cites ways to tell if you need OPC: "In the morning you brush your teeth and discover that your gums are bleeding. Or you notice a speck of blood on the cornea of the eye. Or at night you feel tired, your calves are swollen, you notice edema. In that case you're suffering from vascular fragility, and OPC fights all these pathological mechanisms."

Europeans for forty years have benefited from OPC treatment to relieve capillary and circulatory disorders, primarily varicose veins. And the research, much of it done by Dr. Masquelier and colleagues, is compelling. In 1995 a major review of the research by Italian investigators concluded that OPC indeed worked, sometimes better than other potent human-made pharmaceutical drugs. One 1981 well-conducted (double-blind) study of fifty patients with varicose veins found that 150 milligrams a day of grape seed OPC (Endotelon) worked faster and longer than a commonly prescribed pharmaceutical drug (Diosmine) in reducing pain, sensations of burning and tingling, and the degree of distention of the veins. All symptoms improved within thirty days. In another study, giving patients with widespread varicose veins just a single 150 milligram dose of OPC improved the tone of their veins, as meticulously measured by a standard test. Another 1985 double-blind controlled study of ninety-two French patients with "venous insufficiency" (varicose veins) showed that 300 milligrams of grape seed OPC daily for twenty-eight days reduced pain, tingling, night leg cramps, and swelling by more than 50 percent. Seventy-five percent of the patients improved on the grape seed medication, making it twice as effective as the dummy pill.

Diffuses High Blood Pressure: OPC may help reverse high blood pressure and its consequences. People with high blood pressure commonly have weakened capillaries with high permeability, boost-

ing their chances of hemorrhagic stroke and ruptured blood vessels in the retina of the eye, research
shows. In animals prone to high blood pressure, OPC
has strengthened capillaries, according to extensive
studies by one of Hungary's most distinguished scientists, Dr. Miklos Gabor. In human terms this
means OPC might keep blood vessels in the brain
and eyes from weakening enough to burst, he says.
Indeed, French researchers have found that grape
seed OPC increased capillary resistance by 25 percent in patients with high blood pressure and/or diabetes, compared with those taking a placebo sugar
pill. Exciting new research by Professor Peter
Rohdewald, a leading pharmaceutical researcher at
the University of Münster in Germany, shows that
pine bark OPC reduces adrenaline stress reactions
that trigger high blood pressure. In animals, brain
damage from strokes was much less in those first
given OPC.

In a particularly convincing demonstration of
OPC's ability to increase capillary "resistance" or
strength, Dr. Rohdewald and colleagues applied a vacuum to the skin of elderly people, which readily produced microbleedings within the skin. But after the
subjects took a single dose of 100 milligrams of pine
bark OPC (Pycnogenol), the vacuum power had to be
increased markedly to produce the microbleeding.
This means the OPC strengthened the capillaries so
"they don't 'leak' or bleed as easily," said Professor
Rohdewald.

Further, it is well known that inflammation and

diabetes abnormally increase the permeability of blood vessels. Giving animals OPC blocked such detrimental increased permeability of brain capillaries, the aorta of the heart, and cardiac muscle capillaries, according to French scientists at the University of Paris.

Fights Cholesterol: Since OPC is an antioxidant, research shows it fights cholesterol by discouraging deposits from forming on artery walls. OPC also corrects dangerous blood-clotting tendencies that trigger heart attacks and strokes. Dr. Ronald Watson, a researcher at the University of Arizona, recently confirmed that OPC (Pycnogenol) normalizes platelet aggregation—blood stickiness leading to hazardous blood clots. He showed that when people smoked, their platelets clumped together in a tendency to form clots. But about twenty minutes after taking OPC, their platelets returned to normal.

How Does It Work?

OPC's main claim to fame is its unique ability to strengthen the walls of blood vessels weakened by age and disease. OPC thus reverses the fragility of blood vessels, making them more intact and supple so blood flows through easily and doesn't leak out. OPC accomplishes this by actually creating tougher, thicker, more tightly knit blood vessel walls that are less apt to stretch, leak, or burst. As Dr. Masquelier explains, two proteins in the vessel wall, collagen and elastin, greatly determine the elasticity and permeability of the vascular wall, whether the wall is solid, strong, and flexible, or fragile and leaky. OPC attaches to these two building block proteins, preventing their degradation by destructive enzymes and encouraging their synthesis and maturation. In short, OPC reinforces the structure of the connective tissue that makes blood vessels strong and resistant.

Part of OPC's power in protecting blood vessels is its anti-inflammatory activity; inflammation is increasingly recognized as contributing greatly to the degradation of arteries and veins. OPC also acts as an antihistamine by blocking the activation of enzymes that regulate histamine release. "Although OPC was never released as a pharmaceutical antihistamine, it performs just as well," says Dr. Masquelier.

Should You Try It?

If you think your blood vessels need help—undeniably blood vessels weaken with age and disease—taking OPC could be a smart idea, especially if you are older or concerned about varicose veins, spider veins, age-related deterioration in vision, swelling and edema, allergies, high blood pressure, a tendency to bleed and bruise easily, or a family or personal history of a bleeding stroke or diabetes (a disorder in which blood vessels are more permeable). There is no safe alternative, nothing comparable among other natural remedies, over-the-counter drugs, or even prescription drugs. OPC is safe and relatively inexpensive and could add a whole new dimension of health to a body with a poor and deteriorating circulatory system. Just think, if OPC reinforces the walls of any blood vessel, it does the same for all arteries, veins, and capillaries. It is not selective. The potential payoff is enormous in fighting vascular disease in all its destructive guises.

How Much? Recommended therapeutic doses of OPC are between 150 and 300 milligrams daily to treat illnesses, and between 50 and 100 milligrams to maintain good vascular health.

Safety: OPCs are expected to be safe because they are widespread in the food supply; however, they have been tested for toxicity in laboratory mice, rats, guinea pigs, and dogs, and have been declared nontoxic, nonmutagenic, noncarcinogenic, and free of side effects, according to a review of the evidence by German researcher Professor Peter Rohdewald. Additionally, in tests of OPC on humans, doctors have not reported adverse effects, say experts.

Which to Take? Commercially, you can get OPC as a grape seed extract or a pine bark extract known as Pycnogenol, a brand name. Unfortunately, not all grape seed products are created equal, and it's difficult for consumers to know how much OPC is actually in a given brand. There are at least two well-known reputable brands. The grape seed pharmaceutical quality extract, known as Endotelon in Europe and thoroughly tested there as a treatment for varicose veins and other vascular diseases, is being sold in the

United States by Nature's Way as Dr. Jack
Masquelier's Tru-OPCs, and by NaturaLife as Dr. Jack
Masquelier's Authentic OPCs. Pycnogenol™ (made
in France) is marketed in this country by Henkel
Corporation, the well-respected U.S. supplement
maker. Both are high quality, although Pycnogenol is
more expensive.

Chapter 10

Fabulous Fish Oil— The Omega-3s

It can fix up your heart and blood. It's a unique and potent medicine.

Your heart rhythm is abnormal, making you vulnerable to sudden death from heart attack. Your blood triglycerides are too high or your blood vessels are slightly clogged and you're afraid an artery may clamp shut, triggering a heart attack or stroke. You've already had one heart attack and fear you may have another. You may need one of nature's most marvelous, versatile medicines—those unique fatty molecules found in fish. An earlier chapter described the effects of eating fish-rich diets; here you'll see the benefits of supplementing with fish oil capsules.

Remarkable new research is finding that this peculiar type of fat is so essential to your cells that they malfunction without it. The reason: Fish oil, along with other types of fat in the membranes encapsulating cells, literally controls the cell's behavior. And as each cell goes, so goes the rest of the body. A minuscule imbalance of fatty acids in individual cells can make them go berserk, creating chaos throughout your body.

Only in the last decade have scientists begun to understand how the fat content of cells can foster illness and how infusing cells with the right fat can correct the fatty imbalance, making dysfunctional cells behave properly and disease symptoms subside. Among other things, the omega-3 fatty acids in fish temper our cells' angry inflammatory attacks on other cells, keep cell membranes pliable enough to slip easily through blood vessels, rev up antioxidant defenses, and modulate the passage of electrochemical messages through heart cells. Leading scientists throughout the world acknowledge that fish oil is a therapeutic wizard, full of surprises.

What Is It?

The particular type of fatty acid in fish oil is unique. It is called long-chain omega-3. Some plant foods— rapeseed (canola oil), flaxseed, walnuts—also have omega-3s that are not as potent as those in fish. Additionally, fish oil or omega-3s are of two types— EPA, long touted as crucial in heart disease; and DHA, now known to be important in brain functions. You get these fish oils when you eat fatty fish, such as mackerel, sardines, salmon, and herring. Fish oil, containing specific amounts of omega-3 fatty acids, is also put into soft-gel capsules that you can take therapeutically.

The Evidence

Lessens Heart Attack Risk: It's a good idea to eat fish to ward off a first heart attack, and eating fish may even help keep you safe from subsequent attacks. But it's much more reliable to take fish oil capsules, especially if you're not a fish lover, and it's all the more critical if you have already suffered a heart attack.

Proof comes in a striking new large-scale, first-of-its-kind Italian study. Franco Valagussea and colleagues in Milan have found that taking only 1,000 milligrams of fish oil capsules every day slashed the risk of death by 20 percent over the next few years following a heart attack. In this study, 11,324 heart attack victims were followed for three and a half years. One-fourth of them took fish oil capsules, one-fourth took 300 milligrams of vitamin E daily, one-fourth took both, and one-fourth took none. Surprisingly, the fish oil capsules were more effective than vitamin E in warding off future deadly heart attacks.

Unclogs Arteries: Several studies have suggested that taking fish oil capsules prior to and after angioplasty (surgery to open narrowed arteries) may reduce the amount of reclosure in the arteries. For example, a review in 1993 of research by investigators at the Medical College of Wisconsin identified seven studies that noted a slower reclosure rate of arteries when patients took fish oil. Further, the higher the doses of fish oil the greater the success. In one study the rate of reclogging was slowed down by 24 percent. However, a subsequent study did not show such dramatic benefits of taking fish oil capsules in keeping arteries open after surgery. Why it worked in some and not others is unknown.

Quells Arrhythmias: If you have heart disease and are at high risk of cardiac arrhythmias—irregular heartbeats—that can trigger sudden death, you should be sure to get sufficient fish oil. New research suggests that fish oil can help keep heart rhythms from going berserk.

About a quarter of a million Americans die suddenly each year when their hearts abruptly go into a fatal arrhythmia. It happens because the electrical transmission of impulses that govern the rate or rhythm of the heartbeat goes haywire. Although it can strike anyone out of the blue, people who have had heart attacks are at especially high risk. Now remarkable new research suggests that fish oil may be a marvelous medicine to help regulate heart rhythms, preventing fatal cardiac arrhythmias. Such a promising role for fish oil is entirely new. Although researchers have known for years that eating fatty fish helps prevent heart disease, and notably death from heart disease, it was thought that fish oil acted mostly by protecting the arteries against plaque buildup and by thinning the blood. Now researchers suspect that the most profound benefits from fish oil come from directly protecting the heart against electrical malfunction leading to sudden death.

As mentioned earlier in this book (page 14), fish oil affects the electrical activity and "excitability" of heart cells. To recap: Harvard researcher Dr.

Alexander Leaf has shown that it is much more difficult to induce heart arrhythmias in dogs that are first
given fish oil. It took a 50 percent stronger electrical
stimulus to induce cardiac arrythmias in heart cells
that contained high levels of omega-3 fatty acids. Dr.
Leaf is now testing the theory in humans; results are
still not out. In his study, patients with implanted
defibrillators who have already had heart attacks will
take either fish oil capsules or olive oil capsules for a
year. The study will reveal whether fish oil reduces the
number of times the defibrillator must discharge to
correct a heart arrhythmia.

At least two major studies, in England and France,
tend to indirectly confirm the therapeutic ability of
omega-3 fat to suppress fatal arrhythmias after a heart
attack. In studies of about 1,600 patients, those who
ate omega-3 as fatty fish, fish oil capsules, or canola
oil were much less apt to suffer subsequent fatal heart
attacks (not necessarily nonfatal heart attacks) than
those not taking in high omega-3. In fact, in one
study not a single patient on high omega-3s died of
cardiac arrest. Also, direct support for the idea comes
from a new study in Denmark of fifty-five heart attack
patients. Half took fish oil capsules (5 grams, or about
fifteen capsules a day) for three months. The fish oil
affected their hearts in ways that inhibited deadly cardiac

What's most remarkable, says Dr. Leaf, is that
omega-3 "medication" appears to give rapid protection against cardiac sudden death. Researchers have
noticed a reduction in cardiac deaths within a month

of increased intakes of omega-3 fatty acids. Compare that with the two or three years needed to reap the heart attack protection of lowering your blood cholesterol. This newly discovered direct effect of omega-3s on heart function also helps explain why fish eaters have fewer heart attacks and are less apt to die from them.

Further, new evidence reveals that fish oil, like vitamin C, influences all-important vascular function, keeping arteries more relaxed and open so blood can flow through. The omega-3s, like the vitamin, somehow trigger release of nitric oxide, the chemical that tells artery walls to relax.

Certainly, anyone who has ever had a heart attack—or who has signs of heart disease—should seriously consider fish oil an essential medication that could be lifesaving, particularly by suppressing deadly fibrillation if a heart attack occurs.

Smashes Triglycerides: Fish oil can curb heart disease in other ways. In fact, it is almost a sure cure—*better than any known drug*—for high triglycerides, a type of blood fat that can be dangerous to arteries, especially when coupled with low good type HDL cholesterol. In fact, fish oil is probably the safest and best "drug" around for reducing triglycerides, according to a new analysis of the data by William Harris, Ph.D., director of the Lipoprotein Research Laboratory, Mid America Heart Institute of St. Luke's Hospital in Kansas City. Dr. Harris reviewed seventy-two well-controlled human studies and found that fish oil supplements reduced abnormally high triglycerides an average of 28 percent in patients. The effective fish oil dose was 3,000 to 4,000 milligrams daily, which is ten to thirteen capsules of the 300 milligram capsules commonly available in health food stores. New high-potency fish oil capsules also available, which cuts the number down to three or four capsules and are sold through some pharmacies. You can count on fish oil to work quickly; triglycerides start to sink in a few days and hit normal within a couple of weeks.

A possible drawback: Fish oil typically raises bad LDL cholesterol slightly, discouraging some doctors from recommending the oil to reduce triglycerides. Dr. Harris does not find this worrisome, but Canadian researchers have come up with a solution: also take garlic. In a recent study, when men took 900 milligrams of garlic powder daily along with fish oil capsules, triglycerides fell 34 percent and LDL cholesterol dropped 9.5 percent. The senior author, Bruce J. Holub of the University of Guelph in Ontario, urges trying "effective and safe" combination before resorting to expensive prescription drugs to lower triglycerides and cholesterol.

The triglyceride-lowering alternative: very high doses of niacin or prescription drugs, all with potentially hazardous side effects.

Lowers Blood Pressure: Several studies attest to this. For example, German research by Dr. Peter Singer found small doses of fish oil as effective in reducing blood pressure as the beta-blocker Inderal, a commonly prescribed blood pressure medication, as he reported at the 1990 International Conference on

Fish Oils in Washington, D.C. He also found that Inderal and fish oil together reduced blood pressure better than either did alone. University of Cincinnati tests found that blood pressure fell 4.4 points diastolic and 6.5 points systolic in subjects with mild blood pressure who took 2,000 milligrams of omega-3 fatty acids daily for three months. The drop was enough to eliminate the need for medication in some people.

How Does It Work?

Astounding as it may seem, the type of fatty acids in your cells orchestrate a myriad of events that determine your well-being. Most critical is the balance of types of fatty acids in cells. Too much of one type of oil, called omega-6 (dominant in corn oil, for example), causes them to spew off inflammatory chemicals that stab pains into your joints and inflame the inner lining of your intestinal tract. Whereas omega-3 oil, dominant in fish, tends to subdue inflammation—a process underlying disease. Fish oil also spurs release of chemicals that can influence electrical activity in the heart.

How Much? The precise dose of omega-3s needed to ward off heart attacks is not known, although much research indicates that most healthy people probably can get enough omega-3 to their hearts and arteries by eating oily fish, such as salmon, mackerel, sardines, herring, and anchovies two or three times a week. However, if you don't like fish, can't eat that much, have had a heart attack, or are at high risk of heart disease or need therapeutic doses, fish oil capsules are the answer. Indeed, some researchers think most Americans could benefit from taking one or two standard fish oil capsules a day—a dose of 300 to 600 milligrams of omega-3 fatty acids, to fight artery clogging and possibly prevent heart stoppage. Some capsules now have a higher content of omega-3s (EPA and DHA), so check the label.

Safety: If you are on anticoagulants or blood thinners such as Coumadin, consult your doctor about taking fish oil supplements.

Some fears have been expressed over the possibility of excessive oxidation (cell-destroying free radicals) and environmental contaminants, such as pesticides and mercury, in fish oil capsules. However, Harvard's Dr. Leaf, who takes fish oil capsules himself, says he considers the capsules safe—in fact, safer than eating certain fish; for example, those from contaminated inland waters. He says responsible processors do meticulously "cleanse" the fish oils to be put in capsules of hazardous agents and add vitamin E to inhibit oxidation. (Be sure the capsule contains vitamin E, which will be noted on the label.) One way to determine a good quality pure fish oil capsule, says one industry expert, is by the light color of the oil. He suggests laying different brands of fish oil capsules on a white piece of paper and choosing the capsule that appears lightest. Also, if a fish oil capsule has a strong fish odor and taste, you should reject it for one that tastes fresh.

Caution: Always store fish oil capsules, or any capsules of vegetable oils, in the refrigerator. Lower temperatures can slow down the rate at which they turn rancid; rancidity is the same as oxidation, or the generation of dangerous free radical chemicals that promote all types of chronic diseases.

Interfering Factor: Too much of a type of fat called omega-6 can sabotage the benefits of fish oil. This omega-6 fat is found in vegetable oils, primarily corn oil, regular safflower and sunflower seed oil, and products made with them, such as mayonnaise, shortenings, and salad oils. Animal fat in meat and dairy foods can also overwhelm the omega-3 fat in cells, throwing things out of whack. To get the full benefit of fish oil, in food or capsules, you must also cut down on animal fats and omega-6 fats.

Chapter 11

Garlic the Great

Garlic is one of nature's heart wonder drugs, whether taken as food or pills. If you don't like garlic, don't want garlic breath, or reject fresh garlic for other reasons, take garlic supplements.

To safeguard your heart and live a longer, more vital life, feed your cells that ancient medicinal herb, garlic—revered for nearly five thousand years as a health tonic and virtual cure-all. Science now is beginning to understand how garlic works. The bulb is packed with at least four hundred chemicals, including many antioxidants, that guard cells from damage, protect arteries, promote blood flow, and retard aging. Supplements made from garlic have been shown to help combat cardiovascular disease.

The Evidence

Lowers Cholesterol: Garlic supplements lower high cholesterol (over 200) an average 23 points, or about 9 percent, according to a major review of the evidence by Stephen Warshafsky at New York Medical College in Valhalla, New York. His analysis

Garlic's Active Compounds

Garlic contains dozens of therapeutic compounds; here are the most important:

Alliin: Its chemical name is S-allylcysteine sulfoxide, an odorless sulfur amino acid derivative found inside the garlic bulb. As soon as the bulb is ruptured by cutting or crushing, alliin is quickly converted into allicin by enzymes.

Allicin: This is the sulfur compound that imparts a fresh garlic odor. Cooking destroys allicin but releases other agents, such as ajoene and adenosine, that act as anticoagulants. Thus, raw and cooked garlic have different medicinal properties.

Ajoene: Named for the Spanish word for garlic, *ajo*, this sulfur-containing compound is formed minutes after crushing or mincing raw garlic. Plays a role in cholesterol lowering and clot prevention.

Sulfur-Containing Amino Acids: Less odiferous than some of garlic's other compounds, they trigger antioxidant systems and lower cholesterol production in the body. Examples: S-allylcysteine and gamma-glutamyl-S-allylcysteine.

"Organic Sulfide" Compounds: Diallyl disulfide and methyl allyl sulfide have anticholesterol and anticancer properties.

included tests of a daily 900 milligrams of Kwai garlic powder tablets, a spray-dried powder, and 1,000 milligrams of Kyolic water extract. Amazingly, the studies suggest that a couple of cloves of garlic or the equivalent in supplements may be as potent as cholesterol-lowering drugs that are deemed effective if they reduce cholesterol 15 percent. You need to take garlic for over a month to get cholesterol-lowering benefits. A similar British meta-analysis, or statistical analysis, of other data found an average cholesterol reduction of 12 percent from garlic supplements.

Garlic compounds actually stop the body from manufacturing cholesterol, according to new research from the University of Pennsylvania. Cholesterol is synthesized in the liver; thus, researchers injected liver cells with a variety of garlic compounds to determine their effect on cholesterol production. While many suppressed cholesterol synthesis to some degree, three compounds, including S-allylcysteine, suppressed it by a whopping 40 to 60 percent!

German researchers at the University of Munich isolated six chemicals in garlic that lower blood cholesterol much the same way the cholesterol-lowering drug Mevacor does, by blocking the liver's production of cholesterol. The garlic suppressed cholesterol synthesis by about 50 percent in test animals. One of garlic's strongest anticholesterol substances was ajoene, a compound that also helps deter blood clots and is found in both raw and cooked garlic.

Controversy: In 1998 a widely reported German study cast doubt on garlic's cholesterol-lowering powers. For three months, twenty-eight people with high average cholesterol of 274 (200 or under is ideal) took 900 milligrams of Kwai garlic powder capsules daily (equivalent to about a clove of fresh garlic). Another group took a placebo (dummy pill). Neither group saw a drop in cholesterol levels. However, scientists in the know about garlic say this one dissenting study does not refute garlic's cholesterol-lowering abilities, especially when confronted with overwhelming evidence to the contrary. "The preponderance of the evidence still suggests that garlic does lower cholesterol," affirms University of Pennsylvania garlic researcher Dr. John Milner. Several factors may be responsible for the German anomaly, he explains. For example, the small sample of individuals may have been genetically unresponsive to garlic (it doesn't work on everyone) or the type of garlic preparation was ineffective. "Looking at the totality of the information, garlic lowers cholesterol by 7 to 15 percent," states Dr. Milner.

Detoxifies Cholesterol: Especially crucial is garlic's antioxidant powers to block free radicals from oxidizing bad type LDL cholesterol, thus crippling its ability to clog arteries. In a study by William Harris at the University of Kansas Medical Center, taking six 100 milligram capsules of garlic powder (Kwai) every day for two weeks reduced oxidation of LDL cholesterol by a remarkable 34 percent. This means that although you have high cholesterol, eating garlic tends to neutralize its artery-clogging dangers.

Brings Down Blood Pressure: An analysis of eight controlled studies found that taking 600 to 900 milligrams of Kwai daily (equal to one or two fresh garlic cloves) lowered mild blood pressure an average 8 percent in one to three months, according to Professors Christopher Silagy, University of South Australia, and Dr. Andrew Neil, Oxford University. Further, garlic lowers blood pressure. In one double-blind

The Prozac of the Supermarket?

Since stress contributes to heart disease, anything that reduces stress helps save your heart. "I suspect garlic is antistress, antianxiety and acts as a sort of antidepressant like Prozac, although with a much milder effect," says Dr. Gilles Fillion of the Pasteur Institute in France. "Eating garlic may just make you feel better."

Dr. Fillion found that garlic affects the release of serotonin—a brain chemical involved in regulating a wide spectrum of moods and behavior, including anxiety, depression, pain, aggression, stress, sleep, and memory. Higher levels of serotonin and serotonin activity in the brain tend to act as a tranquilizer to calm you down, induce sleep, and relieve depression. Dr. Fillion believes garlic helps normalize the serotonin system. A Japanese study of mice once found that garlic extract was 60 percent as effective as Valium in relieving stress.

German study, taking supplements equaling two garlic cloves daily reduced blood pressure from 171/102 to 152/89 after three months.

Fights Clots: Another critical way garlic fights heart disease is by discouraging formation of dangerous clots, or "thinning the blood." Garlic blocks blood platelets from sticking to each other or the walls of arteries, a first step to artery clogging. Eric Block, professor of chemistry at the State University of New York at Albany, has isolated ajoene, the garlic chemical with anticoagulant activity equal or superior to that of aspirin. Garlic also revs up the clot-dissolving fibrinolytic system. Three cloves of raw garlic a day improved clot-dissolving activity about 20 percent in a double-blind study of Indian medical students. Cooked garlic seems to have even more antithrombotic activity.

Stops Heart Attacks: Even after you have heart disease or a heart attack, eating or taking garlic may help save you. Pioneering garlic researcher and cardiologist Arun Bordia at Tagore Medical College in India says garlic seems to help dissolve blockages in arteries, partially "healing" arteries damaged by atherosclerosis. Dr. Bordia has found that feeding garlic to rabbits with severe atherosclerosis reduced the degree of blockage in their arteries. More remarkably, he documented that eating garlic after a heart attack helped prevent subsequent heart attacks and deaths. In his study of 432 heart attack patients, those who ate two or three fresh garlic cloves— raw or cooked—every day suffered only half as many fatalities after two years as those eating no garlic. The benefits were more impressive after three years. During that time, garlic eaters suffered only one-third as many deaths and nonfatal heart attacks as non-garlic eaters.

Dr. Bordia suggests that since the benefits of garlic increased with time, the most plausible explanation is a shrinkage in blockages of coronary arteries.

Garlic also fights aging and clogging in peripheral arteries as well as heart arteries. It can relieve intermittent claudication (pains in legs due to a blockage or narrowing of leg arteries). After taking garlic powder (Kwai, 800 milligrams daily), patients with intermittent claudication were able to walk fifty yards farther without stopping than those on a placebo could. Usually victims can walk only short distances at a time because of cramplike pain in the legs. The improvement occurred after five weeks of garlic treatment, according to German researchers.

How Does It Work?

Garlic is an incredibly complex mixture of chemicals, and scientists are still baffled by which substances have the most profound effects on the heart. But it is known that garlic chemicals have a range of talents—as cholesterol reducers, anticoagulants, blood pressure reducers, and anti-inflammatory agents—all of which affect the heart.

Some research suggests that garlic behaves much like a class of prescription blood pressure drugs called angiotensin-converting enzymes, or so-called ACE inhibitors. In fact, garlic compounds have been patented as ACE inhibitors to lower blood pressure. Garlic extract has also been found to have beta-blocker activity by decreasing the strength and frequency of vascular muscle contractions. Beta-blockers are well-known heart and blood pressure drugs.

Garlic Supplements

Many garlic supplements are on the market. Here are the main claims of the leading brands:

Kwai: A German-made dried garlic preparation that bases most of its health claims on its "allicin potential"; in other words, it releases allicin. It is coated and dissolves in the intestinal tract, not in the stomach, which may help reduce garlic breath and stomach irritation.

Kyolic: A Japanese "aged garlic extract" that does not contain allicin. It comes in liquid (aged in alcohol) or dried powder, and is full of sulfur-containing compounds. It has a standardized amount of one of garlic's pharmacologically active chemicals, such as S-allylcysteine.

Garlic powder: This is the same stuff that's on your spice rack. Raw garlic is dried and processed. Analyses have shown it may contain lots of allicin, but since it is not standardized for content of allicin or sulfur compounds as are traditional garlic supplements, it's impossible to tell how much is in supermarket batches. It depends on the richness of the garlic used, which can vary greatly.

Garlic oil supplement: A distillation of garlic or garlic extracts that is diluted in vegetable oil. Depending on how garlic is processed, it produces a unique brew of chemicals, so you can't be sure what type of doses you're getting.

How much? In supplements, 600 to 900 milligrams of active garlic powder per day has produced documented heart-protective effects. (For fresh or cooked garlic, half a clove to two or three a day should give your cells a heart-defending injection.)

How Potent? The potency of garlic depends on the size of the clove and the soil in which it is grown. Here's a rough guide to equivalent doses found in fresh garlic cloves, powder, and pills:

Two or three fresh garlic cloves equal one teaspoon of garlic powder (the stuff you find on the spice rack); four one-gram (1,000 milligrams) powdered garlic tablets, such as Kwai; four gel caps of Kyolic garlic; or one teaspoon of liquid Kyolic garlic.

Safety: Don't exceed the manufacturers recommended doses; too much garlic can irritate the stomach and may even be toxic.

Food vs. Pills: In most aspects (but probably not all), garlic supplements contain the same protective chemicals as fresh garlic. Such supplements have been widely tested in animals and humans, especially in Germany, Japan, and the United States, and exhibited definite cardiovascular benefits. Garlic pills are the best-selling over-the-counter drug in Germany. And many researchers in the United States say they regularly take garlic supplements as well as eat fresh garlic.

Chapter 12

Fiber Zaps Cholesterol, Unclogs Arteries

It promises to lower your cholesterol more dramatically than anything else you can take, and it may clean out your arteries, too—all without the side effects of drugs.

It starts in childhood and progresses relentlessly until your arteries are wrecked—stiff, hard, and stuffed with plaque and debris. By middle age, most of us are hoping for a medical miracle to rescue us from the dreaded consequences of this premier killer, atherosclerosis. True, with a strict diet, drugs, exercise, and stress control, you may be able to stop the damage to your arteries from progressing. But what if you could swallow a powder to significantly reopen clogged arteries so blood can better flow through to the heart and brain, lessening your chances of heart attacks, bypass surgery, strokes, chest pain, and all the ills brought on by clogged arteries? And how about driving down cholesterol, when even the latest brainchild of the pharmaceutical industry has failed to work?

There is such a powder that more than one user has dubbed a miracle. It's a special grapefruit fiber mixture, a unique form of pectin—a water-soluble fiber—obtained mostly from the rinds, membranes, and juice sacs of the grapefruit, and combined with another soluble fiber, guar gum. It is processed into a pale yellow, tasteless powder to be dissolved in liquids or sprinkled on food. It is patented by the University of Florida and by Dr. James Cerda and is commercially called ProFibe.

The Evidence

Literally dozens of excellent studies in the United States and elsewhere have found that soluble fiber and its by-products in various foods, including beta glucans in oats and pectin in fruit, can all lower blood cholesterol. Following that lead, Dr. James J. Cerda, a gastroenterologist and professor of medicine at the University of Florida College of Medicine, for twenty years has focused on the unique powers of pectin, a soluble fiber in grapefruit, to save and restore arteries. Dr. Cerda's first breakthrough experiment in 1988 showed that grapefruit pectin dramatically lowered cholesterol in miniature pigs put on a high-fat diet. The pig's cardiovascular system is almost identical to that of a human. Cerda fed the pigs a diet with 15 percent lard (equal to about 40 percent of calories in fat). Predictably, their cholesterol soared and their arteries closed. But when the pigs also ate pectin, their blood cholesterol fell 20 to 25 percent. Still, that was not the biggest surprise. When Dr. Cerda examined their arteries under the microscope, he was incredulous.

The arteries of the pectin-fed pigs were much less clogged and generally much healthier.

Dr. Cerda suspected that grapefruit pectin, regardless of lowering cholesterol, could also prevent and even reverse artery clogging. So for another year, fifteen new pigs were fed lots of lard. Then Dr. Cerda added grapefruit fiber to half the pigs' fatty diets. Nine months later the pigs were sacrificed and their arteries and hearts painstakingly examined. "It was so exciting," exclaims Dr. Cerda. The arteries of the pigs fed pectin were much healthier, revealing little of the destruction to arteries found in pigs not fed pectin— the hunks of plaque stuck in artery walls and narrowed arteries able to accommodate only trickles of blood. The researchers measured the amount of arterial surface area covered by plaque and diameters of arterial openings. The astonishing finding: The pectin-fed pigs had fully 60 percent less atherosclerosis in their coronary arteries and aortas. That meant pectin was a remarkable healer of arteries, opening and smoothing them out, or a strong block to the progression of atherosclerosis. Or both.

Everybody's Cholesterol Falls

In humans, Dr. Cerda has documented that ProFibe grapefruit fiber reduces cholesterol in virtually everyone to some degree. In one study he measured the cholesterol of the first 100 patients who consecutively came to the heart clinic at the hospital where he practices. He encouraged all of them to start on 15 grams (about a third of a cup) of the grapefruit fiber daily. "What we found was incredible," says Dr. Cerda. "Their cholesterol, usually in the range of 220 to 300, dropped very quickly as much as 25 to 30 percent in one month!" In some people with exceptionally high cholesterol, grapefruit fiber does reduce it, but not enough to make doctors happy. In such cases a combination of standard cholesterol-lowering drugs, such as Mevacor and Zocor, plus grapefruit fiber may work. A small unpublished study of seven patients with cholesterol of 350 to 400 found that either grapefruit pectin alone or drugs alone brought it down to 225 to 300. On standard doses of both the grapefruit pectin and drugs, the cholesterol frequently dropped below 200.

Human tests of ProFibe's ability to open up arteries, reversing atherosclerosis, are planned on 200 patients with diseased carotid arteries at several centers around the United States. In a double-blind test, half will get real grapefruit fiber (ProFibe) and half will get a lookalike inactive powder (placebo) for eighteen to twenty-four months. Any regression or clearing of the arteries will be detected by ultrasound.

How Does It Work?

The exact mechanisms by which soluble fiber reduces cholesterol are not clear. Some theories: The fiber creates an ultra-thin layer of water in the intestinal tract, hindering absorption of cholesterol-raising fat; the fiber produces by-product chemicals that suppress the liver's production of cholesterol, somewhat the way prescription drugs do. How grapefruit fiber might dissolve plaque buildup and open up arteries is more mysterious. Dr. Cerda speculates that a unique polysaccharide in grapefruit, galacturonic acid, chemically interacts with the destructive stuff in arteries, including bad LDL cholesterol, to prevent and break up plaque deposits.

There's also some evidence that aggressive lowering of cholesterol, as shown with drugs, tends to open arteries, improve blood flow, and cause a regression of atherosclerosis. But Dr. Cerda is convinced that grapefruit fiber's ability to diminish plaque in arteries is independent of its cholesterol-lowering capabilities.

Three Cases of Dramatic Success

Artery Opens, No Need for Surgery

At age 70, S. L. Garrett had little reason to worry about a stroke or heart attack. His blood cholesterol was normal. An exam several years earlier, prompted by slight chest pain, had uncovered no heart problems. Then in December 1994 he had an alarming disturbance of vision in his left eye, signaling a TIA (transient ischemic attack), a common prelude to stroke. Doctors first did a CT scan, finding no brain damage, and then ordered an ultrasound of his carotid arteries, leading up the sides of the neck to the brain. They suspected a blockage. Sure enough, resonating in the left artery was that characteristic sound, or bruit, a distinctive whoosh indicating restricted blood flow. An arteriogram, in which a catheter is inserted at the base of the neck to take X-ray pictures of the carotid arteries, confirmed that Garrett's left carotid artery was 40 percent closed with plaque. And there were signs of ulceration, damage to the artery's interior walls. His right carotid artery was clogged to a lesser extent. The narrowing was not enough to warrant balloon surgery (an endocardectomy) to open it, but it was worrisome. If the artery clogging progressed, the next event could be a full-blown stroke. The recommended therapy: Take anticoagulants to increase blood flow, and medically monitor the condition.

Garrett, fearing the side effects of the anticoagulant, didn't like the idea. And aspirin, another blood-thinning possibility, was out of the question because he was allergic to it.

His son, S. W. "Wayne" Garrett, M.D., a radiologist at Columbia Putnam Medical Center in Patatka, Florida, suggested an alternative. He knew of experiments with grapefruit pectin, a fiber, conducted by Dr. James Cerda at the University of Florida, showing that pectin might clear out arteries. In fact, Cerda had been his professor in medical school. Dr. Garrett also knew the fiber dramatically lowered cholesterol. "Just to show Dad it was okay, I decided to try the pectin myself for a month—and I had a life insurance exam coming up, so I figured, how can it hurt?" said Dr.

Garrett. He also liked the fact that unlike other cholesterol-reducing or cardiac drugs, the fiber has no
dangerous side effects.

So he took Dr. Cerda's grapefruit fiber for a month
and was stunned by the result. "My cholesterol, which
ordinarily runs 180 to 200, dived to 150. More important, my HDLs [good cholesterol] jumped so high,
they surpassed my LDLs [bad cholesterol]. My ratio
was incredible—under one. I was amazed, really
amazed it was that good." (The lower the ratio of
LDLs or total cholesterol to HDLs, the lower the risk
of heart disease. A ratio of under one is highly unusual and protective, especially in men.)

The senior Garrett, impressed, started taking the
grapefruit fiber in January 1995—three times a day,
usually mixed into water or juice. Sixteen months
later, in May 1996, he underwent another ultrasound
examination of his carotid arteries. Their interior
landscape had changed dramatically. The plaque had
shrunk, actually regressed more than one-third—
down from a 40 percent closure to a 25 percent closure in the left carotid artery. The arterial walls, once
bumpy with the plaque's debris, were much smoother
and flatter. The ulceration was almost gone. Because
the opening of the arteries had expanded so much, the
blood flow through the arteries was "excellent."

Where did the plaque go? Obviously, it was somehow dislodged, dissolved, swept away by the action of
the grapefruit fiber. "No question, since Dad did nothing else different, it has to be the fiber," says his son
the physician. Further, the grapefruit fiber surely

helped clear other arteries in the body, because it does not target one specific blood vessel. "I feel more energetic than I've felt in years," says S. L. Garrett.

Is it a miracle? It certainly seems like one to many who use it. Nobody can think of a pharmaceutical drug that could have caused the entrenched plaque to disappear, opening the arteries. The most such drugs do, if you're lucky, is to preserve the status quo so arteries don't get worse. But actually reverse the clogging? Medical consensus says it's unlikely, if not impossible, especially in such a short time and especially with something as benign as grapefruit fiber. Dr. Cerda agrees that "if a new pharmaceutical drug did the same thing—removed one-third of the plaque from old beaten-up arteries, the makers would declare it a miracle cure, sell it for a trillion dollars, and everybody would want it."

A 90-Point Cholesterol Dive in One Month

Joan Levin has a master's degree in public health from Johns Hopkins University as well as a law degree, so when her cholesterol began to climb steadily after age 50, she knew what to do. She went on every cholesterol-controlling regimen she could find. "I tried everything—very rigorous low-fat diets and exercise, but nothing made a dent. I was afraid to take drugs like Mevacor and Zocor because of side effects—liver damage. Anything that affects liver metabolism, as these drugs do, scared me." Still, her cholesterol was going up, up, up, and her physician insisted that cholesterol-lowering drugs were her only option because nothing else worked.

In the summer of 1996 she heard about a special grapefruit fiber product. She started taking it dissolved in water. Although the directions said to take it three times a day, she took it usually twice a day, always being careful to get the full day's recommended dose. After a month she had her blood cholesterol tested. When she got the report in the mail it was so unbelievable, she actually let out a yelp. Her cholesterol had dived from 295 to 208! "The LDL [bad cholesterol] and the triglycerides went down about 100 points. It was just fantastic, really miraculous. I can't see why anyone would want to start hazardous cholesterol drugs before trying this. If it doesn't work after a month, you know it, and can then go on to something else."

"I Gave Up Mevacor for Grapefruit Fiber."

Dr. Daniel Knauf, a vascular surgeon on the faculty of the University of Florida College of Medicine, says that his 76-year-old mother's cholesterol dropped to its lowest point in recent years, below 200, after she took grapefruit fiber. She was able to totally quit her cholesterol-lowering drugs; she had been on cholesterol-lowering Pravachol for five years and Mevacor for six months, and these were not as effective as the grapefruit fiber. Further, Mevacor produced signs of liver damage. She has happily kept her cholesterol down for two years with grapefruit fiber alone, prompting her heart surgeon son to joke that this stuff "could put me out of business."

How Much? The standard dose used in clinical studies is about one-third of a cup a day, or 15 grams of fiber, divided into three doses taken at breakfast, lunch, and dinner. This much may be needed to achieve a regression of plaque in arteries. However, many people get a dramatic cholesterol drop from just 5 grams (one scoop) or 10 grams (two scoops) daily, says Dr. Cerda.

Safety: Many users have gas, especially until they adapt to the high-fiber intake. Also, loose stools are common, and in some cases, diarrhea. You can reduce the dose or start on a lower dose and work up to a larger dose as your body adapts to the high fiber. Because it is a fruit fiber, there is no long-term toxicity.

Caution: If you have heart disease and especially if you are taking heart medications, consult with your doctor about taking ProFibe. Self-medicating for heart disease without professional advice can be dangerous. Note: You cannot get the same benefit from eating lots of grapefruit, because ProFibe is highly concentrated.

Where to Get It: ProFibe grapefruit powder is sold by mail order and generally is not available in health food stores or other retail outlets. To get more information about or to order ProFibe, you can call 800-756-3999. It costs about $60 a month for the maximum dose, or $2 a day.

Appendix

Foods with the Most Heart-Protective Vitamins, Minerals, and Oils

Foods High in Beta Carotene

•	(milligrams per 3 ½ ounces/100 grams)
Apricots, dried	17.6 (about 28 halves)
Peaches, dried	9.2 (about 7 halves)
Sweet potatoes, cooked	8.8 (about ½ cup mashed)
Carrots	7.9 (about 1¼ medium carrots)
Collard greens	5.4 (about ½ cup)
Kale	4.7 (about ⅔ cup, chopped)
Spinach, raw	4.1 (about 1½ cups)
Apricot, raw	3.5 (about 3 medium)
Pumpkin	3.1 (about ½ cup mashed or canned)
Cantaloupe	3.0 (about ⅒ melon)
Squash, winter	2.4 (about ½ cup mashed)
Beet greens	2.2 (about ⅔ cup cooked)
Romaine lettuce	1.9 (equal of 10 leaves)
Grapefruit, pink	1.3 (about ½ grapefruit)
Mango	1.3 (about ½ mango)
Green lettuces	1.2 (about 10 leaves)
Broccoli, cooked	0.7 (about ⅔ cup)
Brussels sprouts	0.5 (about 5 sprouts)

Foods High in Calcium

(milligrams per serving)

Ricotta cheese: ½ cup	337
Parmesan cheese: 1 ounce	336
Milk: 1 cup	300
Calcium-fortified orange juice: 1 cup	300
Mackerel with bones, canned: 3 ounces	263
Yogurt, no fat: 4 ounces	225
Salmon with bones, canned: 3 ounces	191
Collards, frozen, cooked: ½ cup	179
Dried figs: 5 figs	135
Sardines, with bones: 1 ounce	130
Tofu, firm: ½ cup	118
Turnip greens, fresh, cooked: ½ cup	99
Kale, cooked: ½ cup	90
Broccoli, fresh, cooked: ½ cup	89
Okra, frozen, cooked: ½ cup	88
Baked beans: ½ cup	80
Soybeans, cooked: ½ cup	65
Chickpeas, cooked: ½ cup	60
White beans, cooked: ½ cup	45
Pinto beans, cooked: ½ cup	40

Note: All dairy foods are high in calcium. All cheeses average about 200 mg of calcium per ounce, although some are higher, for example, Parmesan and Romano.

Foods High in Folic Acid

(micrograms per serving)

Chicken livers, simmered: ½ cup	539
Bulgur, cooked: ⅔ cup	158

Okra, frozen, cooked: ½ cup	134
Orange juice, fresh or canned: 1 cup	136
Spinach, fresh, cooked: ½ cup	130
White beans, cooked: ½ cup	120
Red kidney beans, cooked: ½ cup	114
Orange juice, frozen, diluted: 1 cup	109
Soybeans, cooked: ½ cup	100
Wheat germ: 1 ounce	100
Asparagus, fresh, cooked: ½ cup	88
Turnip greens, fresh, cooked: ½ cup	85
Avocado, Florida: ½ fruit	81
Brussels sprouts, frozen, cooked: ½ cup	79
Lima beans, dry, cooked: ½ cup	78
Chickpeas, cooked: ½ cup	70
Sunflower seeds: 1 ounce	65
Orange sections: 1 cup	54
Broccoli, fresh, cooked: ½ cup	53
Mustard greens, fresh cooked: ½ cup	51
Beets, fresh, cooked: ½ cup	45
Raspberries, frozen: ½ cup	33

Note: Many cereals also typically have 100 micrograms of folic acid per serving. Product 19, for example, has 400 micrograms. Check cereal labels for content.

Foods High in Potassium

	(milligrams per serving)
Blackstrap molasses: ¼ cup	2,400
Potato, baked: 1 medium	844
Cantaloupe: ½ fruit	825
Avocado, Florida: ½ fruit	742
Beet greens, cooked: ½ cup	654

Peaches, dried: 5 halves	645
Prunes, dried: 10 halves	626
Tomato juice: 1 cup	536
Yogurt, low-fat: 1 cup	530
Snapper: 3½ ounces	522
Lima beans, dried, cooked: ½ cup	517
Salmon: 3½ ounces	490
Soybeans, cooked: ½ cup	486
Swiss chard, cooked: ½ cup	483
Apricots, dried: 10 halves	482
Orange juice, fresh: 1 cup	472
Pumpkin seeds: 2 ounces	458
Sweet potato, cooked: ½ cup	455
Banana: 1 fruit	451
Acorn squash: ½ cup	446
Almonds: 2 ounces	426
Spinach, cooked: ½ cup	419
Herring: 3½ ounces	419
Milk, skim: 1 cup	418
Mackerel: 3½ ounces	406
Peanuts: 2 ounces	400

Foods High in Selenium

	(micrograms in 3½ ounces/100 grams)
Brazil nuts	2,960
Puffed wheat	123
Tuna, light, canned in water	80
canned in oil	76
Tuna, white, canned in water	65
canned in oil	60
Sunflower seeds, roasted	78

Oysters, cooked	72
Chicken liver, cooked	72
Wheat flour, whole grain	71
Clams, canned	49

Note: Organ meats are generally high in selenium, as are whole grains. Most fruits and vegetables are generally low in selenium; the highest is garlic with 14 micrograms per three and a half ounces.

Foods High in Zinc

	(milligrams per serving)
Oysters, smoked: 3 ounce	103
Oysters, raw, without shell: 3 ounces	63
Pot roast, braised: 3 ounces	7
Calf's liver, cooked: 3 ounces	7
Crabmeat, cooked: ½ cup	6
Turkey, dark meat, roasted: 3½ ounces	5
Crabmeat, steamed: 2 medium	4
Pumpkin and squash seeds: 1 ounce	3

Note: Meat and poultry are generally high in zinc. Many cereals have about 4 milligrams of zinc per serving. Check the label.

Foods High in Vitamin C

	(milligrams per serving)
One guava	165
Red sweet pepper: 1 pepper	141
Cantaloupe: ½ fruit	113
Pimientos, canned: 4 ounces	107

Sweet green pepper: 1 pepper	95
Papaya: ½ fruit	94
Strawberries, raw: 1 cup	84
Brussels sprouts: 6 sprouts	78
Grapefruit juice: from 1 fruit	75
Kiwi fruit: 1 fruit	74
Orange: 1 fruit	70
Orange juice, in carton or from concentrate: ½ cup	52
Broccoli: ½ cup cooked	49
Tomato juice: 1 cup	45
Tomatoes, cooked: 1 cup	45
Grapefruit: ½ fruit	42
Broccoli: ½ cup raw	41
Cauliflower, raw: ½ cup	36
Peas, green, raw: ½ cup	31
Kale, cooked: ½ cup	27

Foods High in Vitamin D

(3½ ounces	International Units [IU])
Eel	4,700
Pilchard	1,500
Sardines, fresh	1,500
Herring, fresh	1,000
Salmon, red	800
Salmon, pink	500
Mackerel	500
Salmon, chinook	300
Herring, canned	225
Salmon, chum	200
Tuna	200
Milk (nonfat, low-fat whole)*	100

* 8 fluid ounces.

Foods High in Vitamin E

Vitamin E is fat-soluble and thus is concentrated in vegetable oils, nuts, and seeds. Legumes and brans are also fairly high. Vitamin E is almost nonexistent in animal foods. Although fruits and vegetables are fairly low in vitamin E, they still provide about 11 percent of vitamin E in American diets. About 64 percent comes from oils, margarines, and shortenings, and about 7 percent comes from grains.

	(milligrams per 3½ ounces)
Nuts and Seeds	
Sunflower seeds	52
Walnuts	22
Almonds	21
Filberts (hazelnuts)	21
Cashews	11
Peanuts, roasted	11
Brazil nuts	7
Pecans	2
Brans and Legumes	
Wheat germ	28
Soybeans, dried	20
Rice bran	15
Lima beans, dried	8
Wheat bran	8
Oils	
Wheat germ	250
Soybean	92

Corn	82
Sunflower	63
Safflower	38
Sesame	28
Peanut	24

Types of Fatty Acids in Oils

(percentages)

Oil	Saturated	Monounsaturated	Omega-6	Omega-3
Flax	9	18	16	57
Canola	6	62	22	10
Soy	15	24	54	7
Walnut	16	28	51	5
Olive (extra virgin)	14	77	8	1
Peanut	18	49	33	0
Corn	13	25	61	1
Safflower (regular)	10	13	77	0
Sesame	13	46	41	0
Sunflower (regular)	11	20	69	0

Note: It's easy to see that corn, safflower, and sunflower seed oils have the most omega-6 fatty acids and the least omega-3, making them more hazardous in general. Flax and canola oils have the best ratios of omega-3 to omega-6. Olive oil is highest in heart-protecting monounsaturated fat.

Omega-3 Fatty Acids in Seafood

Fresh or Frozen Fish	(milligrams per 3½ ounces raw)
Roe, finfish, mixed species	2,345
Mackerel, Atlantic	2,299
Herring, Pacific	1,658
Herring, Atlantic	1,571
Mackerel, Pacific and jack	1,441
Sablefish	1,395
Salmon, chinook (king)	1,355
Mackerel, Spanish	1,341
Whitefish, mixed species	1,258
Tuna, bluefin	1,173
Salmon, sockeye (red)	1,172
Salmon, pink	1,005
Turbot, Greenland	919
Shark, mixed species	843
Salmon, coho (silver)	814
Bluefish	771
Bass, striped	754
Smelt, rainbow	693
Oysters, Pacific	688
Swordfish	639
Salmon, chum	627
Wolfish	623
Bass, freshwater, mixed species	595
Seabass, mixed species	595
Trout, rainbow	568
Pompano, Florida	568
Squid, mixed species	488
Shrimp, mixed species	480
Mussels, blue	441

Oysters, Eastern	439
Tilefish	430
Pollock, Atlantic	421
Catfish, channel	373
Lobster, spiny, mixed species	373
Pollock, Alaska (walleye)	372
Crab, snow (queen)	372
Halibut, Atlantic and Pacific	363
Carp	352
Rockfish, Pacific, mixed species	345
Mullet	325
Crab, blue	320
Snapper, mixed species	311
Crab, Dungeness	307
Ocean perch, Atlantic	291
Tuna, skipjack	256
Grouper	256
Whiting, mixed species	224
Tuna, yellowfin	218
Cod, Pacific	215
Scallops, mixed species	198
Haddock	185
Cod, Atlantic	184
Crawfish	173
Octopus	157
Eel, mixed species	147
Clams	142

Canned Fish	(milligrams per 3½ ounces)
Anchovies, canned in olive oil (drained)	2,055
Salmon, pink (including liquid and bones)	1,651
Sardines, Pacific in tomato sauce (drained, without bones)	1,604
Herring, Atlantic, pickled	1,389
Salmon, sockeye (drained, with bones)	1,156
Sardines, Atlantic in soybean oil (drained, with bones)	982
Tuna (albacore), white in water (drained)	706
Tuna, light, in soybean oil (drained)	128
Tuna, light, in water (drained)	111

Source: U.S. Department of Agriculture.

References

Thousands of scientific studies were consulted for this book; thus, it is impossible to list them all. However, here are some of the most important and interesting published scientific sources that are available in medical libraries. The book also contains much unpublished information obtained through interviews with researchers and news reports in scientific publications.

Acheson, R.M.: Does consumption of fruit and vegetables protect against stroke? *The Lancet* 1983; 1191-93.

Albert, C.M., et al.: Fish consumption and risk of sudden cardiac death. *Journal of the American Medical Association* 1998; 279: 23-28.

Alderman, M.H.: Moderate sodium restriction. Do the benefits justify the hazards? *American Journal of Hypertension* 1990; 3: 499-504.

Anderson, J.W.: Serum lipid response of hypercholesterolemic men to single and divided doses of canned beans. *American Journal of Clinical Nutrition* 1990; 51(6): 1013-19.

Anderson, J.W., et al.: Meta-analysis of the effects of soy protein intake on serum lipids. *New England Journal of Medicine* 333(5): 276-82.

Appel, L.J.: A clinical trial of the effects of dietary patterns on blood pressure. *New England Journal of Medicine* 1997; 336: 1117-24.

Auer, W. Hypertension and hyperlipidaemia: garlic helps in mild cases. *British Journal of Clinical Practice Supplement* 1990; 44(8): 3-6.

Bairati, I.: Double blind, randomized, controlled trial of fish oil supplements in prevention of recurrence of stenosis after coronary angioplasty. *Circulation* 1992; 85: 950-56.

Barrie, N.D.: Effects of garlic oil on platelet aggregation, serum lipids and blood pressure in humans. *Journal of Orthomolecular Medicine* 1987; 2(1): 15-21.

Beilin, L.J.: Alcohol and hypertension. *Clinical and Experimental Hypertension Theory and Practice* 1992; A14(1&2): 119-38.

Beilin, L.J.: Alcohol and hypertension—kill or cure? *Journal of Human Hypertension* 1996; 10(suppl 2): S1-S5.

Bulpitt, C.J.: Vitamin C and blood pressure. *Journal of Hypertension* 1990; 12: 1071-75.

Burr, M.L.: Effects of changes in fat, fish, and fibre intakes on death and myocardial reinfarction: death and reinfarction trial (Dart). *The Lancet*, September 1989: 757-61.

Colquhoun, D.M.: Comparison of the effects on lipoproteins and apolipoproteins of a diet high in monounsaturated fatty acids, enriched with avocado and a high-carbohydrate diet. *American Journal of Clinical Nutrition* 1992; 56: 671-77.

Davidson, M.H.: The hypocholesterolemic effects of B-glucan in oatmeal and oat bran. *Journal of the American Medical Association* 1991; 285(14): 1833-39.

Daviglus, M.L., et al.: Fish consumption and the 30-year risk of fatal myocardial infarction. *New England Journal of Medicine* 1997; 336: 1046-53.

De Lorgeril, M., et al.: Mediterranean alpha-linolenic acid-rich diet in secondary prevention of coronary heart disease. *The Lancet* 1994; 343(8911): 1454-59.

De Lorgeril, M., et al.: Mediterranean diet, traditional risk factors, and the rate of cardiovascular complications after myocardial infarction. *Circulation* 1999; 99(6): 779-85.

De Oliveira e Silva, E.R., et al.: Effects of shrimp consumption on plasma lipoproteins. *American Journal of Clinical Nutrition* 1996; 64: 712-17.

Doll, R.: One for the heart. *British Medical Journal* 1997; 315: 1664-68.

Ernst, E.: Plasma fibrinogen—an independent cardiovascular risk factor. *Journal of Internal Medicine* 1990; 227: 365-72.

Ettinger, P.O.: Arrhythmias and "the holiday heart": alcohol associated cardiac rhythm disorders. *American Heart Journal* 1978; 95: 555-62.

Folts, J.B.: Flavonoids in tea but not coffee given by gastric tube inhibit in vivo platelet activity and thrombus formation in stenosed dog coronary arteries. *FASEB Journal* 1996; 10: A793.

Fraser, G.E.: A possible protective effect of nut consumption on risk of coronary heart disease. *Archives of Internal Medicine* 1992; 152: 1416-23.

Gadkari, J.V.: The effect of ingestion of raw garlic on serum cholesterol level, clotting time and fibrinolytic activity in normal subjects. *Journal of Postgraduate Medicine* 1991; 37(3): 128-31.

Gey, K.F.: Inverse correlation between plasma vitamin E and mortality from ischemic heart disease in cross-cultural epidemiology. *American Journal of Clinical Nutrition* 1991; 53(suppl. 1): 326S-34S.

Gillman, Matthew W.: Inverse association of dietary fat with development of ischemic stroke in men. *Journal of the American Medical Association* 1997; 278: 2145-50.

Ginsberg, H.N., et al.: Effects of reducing dietary saturated fatty acids on plasma lipids and lipoproteins in healthy subjects. *Arteriosclerosis, Thrombosis, and Vascular Biology* 1998; 18: 441-49.

Graham, I.M., et al.: Plasma homocysteine as a risk factor for vascular disease. The European Concerted Action Project. *Journal of the American Medical Association* 1997; 277(22): 1775-81.

Gramenzi, A.: Association between certain foods and risk of acute myocardial infarction in women. *British Medical Journal* 1990; 300(6727): 771-73.

Grobbee, D.E.: Coffee, caffeine and cardiovascular disease in men. *New England Journal of Medicine* 1990; 323(15): 1026-32.

Gross, G.: Analysis of the content of the diterpenes cafestol and kahweol in coffee brews. *Food Chemistry Toxicology* 1997; 35(6): 547-54.

Harvard Health Letter: A special report: high blood pressure, 1990. Harvard Medical School, Health Publications Group.

Hermann, W.: The influence of dietary supplementation with omega-3 fatty acids on serum lipids, apolipoproteins, coagulation and fibrinolytic parameters. *Zeitschrift Für Klinische Medizin* 1991; 46(19): 1363-69.

Hillborn, M.: Alcohol abuse and brain infarction. *Annals of Medicine* 1990; 22(5): 347-52.

Hojnacki, J.L.: Effect of drinking pattern on plasma lipoproteins and body weight. *Atherosclerosis* 1991; 88(1): 49-59.

Houwelingen, R.: Effect of a moderate fish intake on blood pressure, bleeding time, hematology, and clinical chemistry in healthy males. *American Journal of Clinical Nutrition* 1987; 46: 424-36.

Howell, W.II.: Plasma lipid and lipoprotein responses to dietary fat and cholesterol: a meta-analysis. *American Journal of Clinical Nutrition* 1997; 65: 1747-64.

Hu, Frank B.: Dietary fat intake and the risk of coronary heart disease in women. *New England Journal of Medicine* 1997; 337: 1491-99.

Hu, Frank B., et al.: Frequent nut consumption and risk of coronary heart disease in women: prospective cohort study. *British Medical Journal* 1998; 317: 1341-45.

Hu, Frank B., et al.: A prospective study of egg consumption and risk of cardiovascular disease in men and women. *Journal of the American Medical Association* 1999; 281(15): 1387-94.

Isaacsohn, J.L., et al.: Garlic powder and plasma lipids and lipoproteins. *Archives of Internal Medicine* 1998; 158: 1189-94.

Jeppesen, J., et al.: Effects of low-fat, high-carbohydrate diets on risk factors for ischemic heart disease in postmenopausal women. *American Journal of Clinical Nutrition* 1997; 65: 1027-33.

Jing, X. Kang, and Alexander Leaf: The cardiac antiar-
rhythmic effects of polyunsaturated fatty acid. *Lipids*
1996; 31: S-41-44.

Kawano, Y., et al.: Effects of magnesium supplementation in
hypertensive patients : Assessment by office, home, and
ambulatory blood pressures. *Hypertension* 1999; 32: 260-65.

Keli, S.O., et al.: Dietary flavonoids, antioxidant vitamins, and incidence of stroke. *Archives of Internal
Medicine* 1996; 154: 637-42.

Khaw, K.: Dietary potassium and stroke associated mortality. *New England Journal of Medicine* 1987; 216: 235-40.

Kiesewetter, H.: Effects of garlic on blood fluidity and
fibrinolytic activity: a randomised placebo-controlled,
double-blind study. *British Journal of Clinical Practice*
1990; 44(suppl. 69)(8): 24-29.

Knapp, H.R.: Omega-3 fatty acids, endogenous
prostaglandins, and blood pressure regulation in
humans. *Nutrition Reviews* 1989; 47(10): 301-13.

Knopp, R.H.: Long-term cholesterol-lowering effects of
4 fat-restricted diets in hypercholesterolemic and
combined hyperlipidemic men. The Dietary
Alternatives Study. *Journal of the American Medical
Association* 1997; 278: 1509-15.

Kohlmeier, L., et al.: Lycopene and myocardial infarction risk in the EURAMIC study. *American Journal of
Epidemiology* 1997; 146: 618-26.

Krauss, R.M.: Understanding the basis for variation in
response to cholesterol-lowering diets. *American
Journal of Clinical Nutrition*, 1997; 65: 885-86.

Krishna, G.C.: Increased blood pressure during potassium depletion in normotensive men. *New England
Journal of Medicine* 1989; 329(18): 1177-82.

Law, M.R.: By how much does dietary salt reduction lower blood pressure? *British Medical Journal* 1991; 302: 819-924.

Leaf, A. Cardiovascular effects of omega-3 fatty acids. *New England Journal of Medicine* 1988; 318: 549-57.

Lipinska, I.: Lipids, lipoproteins, fibrinogen and fibrinolytic activity in angiographically assessed coronary heart disease. *Artery* 1987; 15(1): 44-60.

Lou, F.Q.: A study on tea-pigment in prevention of atherosclerosis. *Chinese Medical Journal* 1989; 102(8): 579-83.

Macko, R.F., et al.: Paper presented at the February 1998 American Heart Association 23rd International Joint Conference on Stroke and Cerebral Circulation.

Makheja, A.: Antiplatelet constituents of garlic and onions. *Agents Actions* 1990; 29(3-4): 360-63.

Malinow, M.R., et al.: Reduction of plasma homocyst(e)ine levels by breakfast cereal fortified with folic acid in patients with coronary heart disease. *New England Journal of Medicine* 1998; 338(15): 1009-15.

Marckmann, P.: Effects of total fat content and fatty acid composition in diet on factor VII coagulant activity and blood lipids. *Atherosclerosis* 1990; 80(3): 227-33.

Margretts, B.M.: Vegetarian diet in mild hypertension: a randomised controlled trial. *British Medical Journal* 1986; 293: 1468-71.

Martin, J.B.: Mortality patterns among hypertensives by reported level of caffeine consumption. *Preventive Medicine* 1988; 17(3): 310-20.

Mehrabian, M.: Dietary regulation of fibrinolytic factors. *Atherosclerosis* 1990; 84: 25-32.

Milner, M.R.: Usefulness of fish oil supplements in preventing clinical evidence of restenosis after percutaneous transluminal coronary angioplasty. *American Journal of Cardiology* 1989; 64(5): 294-99.

Myers, M.G. Coffee and coronary heart disease. *Archives of Internal Medicine* 1992; 152: 1767-72.

Myers, M.G.: Caffeine and cardiac arrhythmias. *Annals of Internal Medicine* 1991; 114: 147-50.

National Institutes of Health, National Heart, Lung and Blood Institute. *Clinical Guidelines on the Identification, Evaluation and Treatment of Overweight and Obesity in Adults: The Evidence Report*. 1998.

Nevill, A.M., et al.: Modelling the associations of BMI physical activity and diet with arterial blood pressure: some results from the Allied Dunbar National Fitness Survey. *Annals of Human Biology* 1997; 24(3): 229-47.

Nygard, O.: Coffee consumption and plasma total homocysteine: The Hordaland Homocysteine Study. *American Journal of Clinical Nutrition* 1997; 65(1): 136-43.

Nygard, O.: Major lifestyle determinants of plasma total homocysteine distribution: the Hordaland Homocysteine Study. *American Journal of Clinical Nutrition* 1998; 67: 263-70.

Omenn, G.S., et al.: Preventing coronary heart disease: B vitamins and homocysteine. *Circulation* 1998; 97: 421-24.

Orlando, J.: Effect of ethanol on angina pectoris. *Annals of Internal Medicine* 1976; 84: 652-55.

Patki, P.S.: Efficacy of potassium and magnesium in essential hypertension: a double-blind, placebo controlled, crossover study. *British Medical Journal* 1990; 301(6751): 521-23.

Peterson, J.C., et al.: Vitamins and progression of atherosclerosis in hyper-homocyst(e)inaemia. *The Lancet* 1998, 351: 263.

Reisin, E.: Effect of weight loss without salt restriction on the reduction of blood pressure in overweight hypertensive patients. *New England Journal of Medicine* 1978; 298: 1-6.

Riemersma, R.A.: Risk of angina pectoris and plasma concentrations of vitamins A, C, and E and carotene. *The Lancet* 1991; 337(8732): 1-5.

Rimm, E.B.: Folate and vitamin B6 from diet and supplements in relation to risk of coronary heart disease among women. *Journal of the American Medical Association* 1998; 279: 359-64.

Ripsin, C.M.: Oat products and lipid lowering: a meta-analysis. *Journal of the American Medical Association* 1992; 267(24): 3317-27.

Robertson, J.: The effect of raw carrot on serum lipids and colon function. *American Journal of Clinical Nutrition* 1979; 32: 1889-92.

Robinson, K., et al. Low circulating folate and vitamin B6 concentrations: risk factors for stroke, peripheral vascular disease, and coronary artery disease. *Circulation* 1998; 97: 437-43.

Sacco, R.L., et al.: The protective effect of moderate alcohol consumption on ischemic stroke. *Journal of the American Medical Association* 1999; 281: 53-60.

Sacks, F.M.: Dietary fats and blood pressure: a critical review of the evidence. *Nutrition Reviews* 1989; 47(10): 291-300.

Sacks, F.: More on chewing the fat. *New England Journal of Medicine* 1991; 325(24): 1740-41.

Sato, Y.: Possible contribution of green tea drinking habits to the prevention of stroke. *Tohoku Journal of Experimental Medicine* 1989; 157(4): 337-43.

Seigneur, M.: Effect of the consumption of alcohol, white wine, and red wine on platelet function and serum lipids. *Journal of Applied Cardiology* 1990; 5: 215-22.

Sendl, A.: Inhibition of cholesterol synthesis in vitro by extracts and isolated compounds prepared from garlic and wild garlic. *Atherosclerosis* 1992; 94(1): 79-85.

Siemann, E.H.: Concentration of the phytoalexin resveratrol in wine. *American Journal of Enol Vitic* 1992; 43(1): 49-52.

Silagy, C.A.: A meta-analysis of the effect of garlic on blood pressure. *Journal of Hypertension* 1994; 12: 463-68.

Simopoulos, A.P.: Omega-3 fatty acids in growth and development and in health and disease. *Nutrition Today*, May/June 1988: 12-18.

Singh, R.B.: Randomized controlled trial of cardioprotective diet in patients with recent acute myocardial infarction: results of one year follow-up. *British Medical Journal* 1992; 304: 1015-19.

Singh, R.B., et al.: Randomized, double-blind, placebo-controlled trial of fish oil and mustard oil in patients with suspected acute myocardial infarction: The Indian experiment of infarct survival-4. *Cardiovascular Drugs and Therapy* 1997; 11: 485-91.

Siscovick, D.S., et al.: Dietary intake and cell membrane levels of long-chain n-3 polyunsaturated fatty acids and the risk of primary cardiac arrest. *Journal of the American Medical Association* 1995; 274: 1363-67.

Spiller, G.A., et al.: Nuts and plasma lipids: an almond-based diet lowers LDL-C while preserving HDL-C. *Journal of the American College of Nutrition* 1998; 17(3): 285-90.

Stampfer, M.: Homocysteine and marginal vitamin deficiency. The importance of adequate vitamin intake. *Journal of the American Medical Association* 1993; 270(22): 2726-27.

Stampfer, M.J.: A prospective study of moderate alcohol consumption and the risk of coronary disease and stroke in women. *New England Journal of Medicine* 319(5): 267-73.

Stefan, K.: Alcohol consumption and atherosclerosis: What is the relation? *Stroke* 1998; 29: 900-7

Steinberg, D.: Alcohol and atherosclerosis. *Annals of Internal Medicine* 1991; 114: 967-76.

Steinberg, D.: Antioxidants in the prevention of human atherosclerosis. *Circulation* 1992; 85(6): 2338-44.

Superko, H.R.: Elevated high-density lipoprotein cholesterol, not protective in the presence of homocysteinemia. *American Journal of Cardiology* 1997; 79(5): 705-6.

Thun, M.J., et al: Alcohol consumption and mortality among middle-aged and elderly U.S. adults. *New England Journal of Medicine* 1997; 337(24): 1705-14.

Tobian, L.: Salt and hypertension. Lessons from animal models that relate to human hypertension. *Hypertension* 1991; 17(suppl. 1): 152-58.

Verlangieri, A.: Effects of d-alpha-tocopherol supplementation on experimentally induced primate atherosclerosis. *Journal of American College of Nutrition* 1992;
11(2): 130-37.

Visudhiphan, S.: The relationship between high fibrinolytic activity and daily capsicum ingestion in Thais.
American Journal of Clinical Nutrition 1982; 35: 1452-
58.

Whelton, P.K.: Sodium reduction and weight loss in the
treatment of hypertension in older persons. *Journal of
the American Medical Association* 1998; 279: 839-46.

Willett, W.C.: Coffee consumption and coronary heart
disease in women. *Journal of the American Medical
Association* 1996; 275: 458-62.

Wilson, P.W.F.: Is coffee consumption a contributor to
cardiovascular disease? *Archives of Internal Medicine*
1989; 149: 1169-72.

Young, W.: Tea and atherosclerosis. *Nature* 1967; 216:
1015-16.

Index

JEAN CARPER is the *New York Times* and national bestselling author *of Miracle Cures, Stop Aging Now!* and *Food: Your Miracle Medicine.* She has a weekly column, "Eat Smart," in *USA Weekend,* which is carried nationally in 550 newspapers, including the *New York Daily News, Denver Post, Chicago Sun-Times, Detroit Free Press,* and *The Minneapolis Tribune.*

YOU *CAN* STOP HEART DISEASE—

While heredity plays a great role in a person's disposition to heart disease, biology can be overcome with the right foods and dietary supplements. *USA Weekend* columnist and number one *New York Times* bestselling author Jean Carper—America's most trusted source of cutting edge nutritional advice—now provides all the information you need to lower the risk of heart disease and its debilitating consequences. *The Miracle Heart* reveals the most current findings available on the remarkable powers of food, vitamins, minerals, and natural remedies that have been shown to prevent, treat, and even reverse heart disease. Here is everything you need to know about:

vitamins E, B, and C • beta carotene • calcium • coenzyme Q-10 • the benefit of superfoods such as fish, garlic, avocados, and strawberries • eggs and cholesterol • the benefits of tea • the secret of olive oil • and much more.

REDUCE BLOOD PRESSURE • LOWER CHOLESTEROL/TRIGLYCERIDES AND HOMOCYSTEINE • AVOID BLOOD CLOTS • HEAL NARROWED ARTERIES • PREVENT STROKES • ENJOY A HEALTHIER LIFE NOW!

This book is largely based on material from Jean Carper's bestselling books *Food—Your Miracle Medicine, Stop Aging Now!,* and *Miracle Cures.*

ISBN 0-06-101383-8

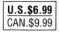

U.S.$6.99
CAN.$9.99